An Incredible Journey

THOMAS Z. LAJOS

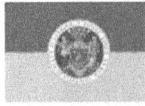

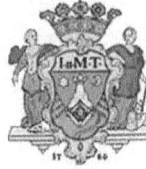

Pècs's flag and coat of arms

My city of birth was Pècs, Hungary. It was an outpost of the Roman Empire: Sopianae. The history of the four-towered cathedral goes back 1,000 years. The first Hungarian University was established at Pècs by King Nagy Lajos in 1342. The city fell to Suleiman the Magnificent after the battle of Mohacs, 1525, and was held for 150 years by the Turks. Pècs received its charter from Marie-Therese, Empress and Kaiserin of the Habsburgs in the late 18th Century. Recently, it was named as one of the cultural capitals of Europe.

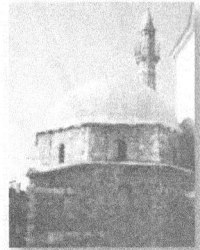

Copyright © 2014 Thomas Z. Lajos. All rights reserved. Barringer Publishing, Naples, Florida. www.barringerpublishing.com. Cover, graphics, layout design by Lisa Camp

ISBN: 978-0-9903935-5-9

Library of Congress Cataloging-in-Publication Data. An Incredible Journey / Thomas Z. Lajos. Printed in U.S.A.

DEDICATION

In memory of my beloved wife,
Charlotte.

TABLE OF CONTENTS

PART I
THE FIRST TWENTY-FIVE YEARS:
OCTOBER 10, 1931- DECEMBER 14, 1956

HUNGARY UNDER NAZI INFLUENCE

THE IRON CURTAIN

PART II
SEARCH FOR ACADEMIC TRAINING IN SURGERY: FREEDOM AND DEMOCRACY: DECEMBER 17, 1956- JULY 1, 1960

THE BRITISH ISLES: LEICESTER AND LONDON, ENGLAND, UK: JAN. 1957-SEPT. 1957

THE NEW WORLD: KINGSTON AND TORONTO, ONTARIO, CANADA

PART III

THE PROFESSIONAL YEARS:
TRAINING IN GENERAL SURGERY

PART IV

THE PROFESSIONAL YEARS:
TRAINING IN CARDIAC AND THORACIC SURGERY

PART V
APPENDICES

LIST OF FIGURES

⁓

Figure 1. My grandfather, Ferenc Lajos, is standing to the right of his father in this photograph taken during the 1890s. My grandfather's three sisters also are shown. The youngest, Ilus, my Grandaunt, sits in the front row.

Figure 2. Taken in the early 1920s, this photograph shows my father, Laszlo, his sister, Jolan, and his brother, Ivan.

Figures 3-5. Top left: Twins, my mother and her brother, Joseph, are shown. Bottom left: Raoul, my maternal grandfather's brother, and Jeno, my maternal grandfather, respectively stand on the left and right. They astonishingly resembled each other. Right: Mr. Raoul Marffy-Mantuano, my maternal grandfather's brother, sits in the sun on the doorstep of his Irmamajor mansion. Pictured respectively in the right and left insets are his wife and his daughter, Judith.

Figure 6. My paternal grandfather, Ferenc Lajos, Principal of the "Realistic School" in Pècs, Hungary.

Figure 7. My father signed this photograph that he gave to my mother, "Don't ever forget me! Laci Dec. 25, 1925."

Figure 8. The front cover of the early English edition of my uncle Dr. Ivan Lajos's book.

Figure 9. I took this photograph in March 1994 while visiting Pècs; my ninety-three year old mother is pictured here with my sister Judy (middle) and my brother Laszlo (far left).

Figure 10. My father walks on the grounds of the Gynecology Hospital in Pècs. The arrows point to the three dining room windows of our flat on the second floor of the hospital.

Figure 11. Another photograph of the Gynecology Hospital in Pècs.

The arrow points to our apartment windows on the second floor.

Figure 12. Professors Elemer Scipiades, Gabor Pal, and Laszlo Lajos are shown from left to right.

Figures 13-14. Top: my maternal grandparents' family cottage at Telep. Bottom: At Telep on Lake Balaton in 1943, my maternal grandparents go for a walk.

Figure 15. Lake Balaton is the second biggest lake in Europe. The line (D4) between Fonyód (on the south shore) and Badacsony (on the north shore) indicates the ferry route.

Figure 16. A photograph of my paternal grandmother taken in the early 1960s.

Figure 17. Mr. József Egry. The Lights of Lake Balaton.

Figure 18. This map of Europe shows the extension and length of the Iron Curtain.

Figures 19-22. The top photograph shows a high-standing border watchtower. The two bottom left diagrams reveal the design of the seventy centimeter barbed wire fences with high posts. The blueprint of the the Iron Curtain is reproduced on the bottom right.

Figure 23. On June 27, 1989, the gates of the Iron Curtain between Hungary and Austria were opened. Memorials were erected at this border.

Figures 24-25. Photographs of the border between West and East Germany: Travemünde, West Germany. The border watchtower, buoys, and signs in the distance demarcated the no man's land or Iron Curtain between the two countries.

Figure 26. Two of my friends stand next to our tent on the shore of the Danube River, on the Baja side in Hungary.

Figure 27. Professor Szilard Donhoffer, Chairman of the Pathophysiology Department at the University of Pècs Medical School, sits at his desk. In his dissertation, which unfortunately never was published, he discussed "Thermoregulation of the Brain."

Figure 28. This stamp was issued in 1967 to commemorate the 600-year anniversary of the founding of the first Hungarian university by King Nagy Lajos. Hungary's first university was founded at Pècs in 1367.

Figure 29. Dean of the University of Pècs Medical School from 1947-1950, my father is pictured here at the age of 42.

Figure 30. This composite picture features faculty members of the University of Pècs's Medical School at the time I graduated in 1956 and during later years, until 1991.

Figures 31-32. These photographs show my father's plaque (top) and the people (bottom) who participated during its unveiling ceremony in October 2011 at the University of Pècs Medical School (POTE). The plaque is affixed to one of the columns in the Aula of the University. Standing from left to right are my sister Judith, Professor Szabo, Department of Gynecology and Obstetrics, my niece Juditka, my brother's wife Agnes, and my brother Laszlo.

Figure 33. Professor József Tigyi is pictured sitting at his desk.

Figure 34. Professor Odon Kerpel-Fronius and his daughter Eva visited Niagara Falls, Ontario, Canada, in the early 1960s.

Figures 35-36. These photographs depict Professor József Kudász (left) and his mentor, Professor Huttle (right). Dr. J. Kudász was a pioneering Hungarian heart surgeon. In the words of Professor Huttle: "One does not become a surgeon, a surgeon is born. One has to learn to see, not only to look. The school of training determines the ability for the surgical technique." Huttle's school provided this opportunity to benefit from these principles.

Figure 37. During the uprisings of October 1956, the demonstrators decapitated and ridiculed Stalin's statue.

Figure 38. The headquarters of the Secret Police (AVO) was taken by the revolutionaries. The captured individuals were hung upside down.

Figure 39. President Carter delivers his "gift," St. Stephen's crown, to the Soviet Chief L. Brezhnev.

Figure 40. The Newman family is pictured from left to right: Frankie, Frank, Johnny, and Jolan; Jolan was my paternal aunt and my godmother.

Figure 41. In this photograph, Dr. Edward H. Simmons is pictured when he was Head of the Department of Orthopedic Surgery at the Buffalo General Hospital and Professor of Orthopedic Surgery at the State University of New York at Buffalo.

Figure 42. A bear rests on the roadside in Yellowstone National Park during the summer of 1960.

Figure 43. Dr. Ed Simmons's Nova Scotia schooner is moored dockside while Ed stands in its cockpit.

Figure 44. This photograph shows a stiffened groundhog in hibernation.

Figure 45. My brother Lacko (standing), Charlotte's sister Cathy (left), Lacko's wife Agnes (middle), and Charlotte (right) while we vacationed in St. Anton, Austria.

Figure 46. I took this photograph of Paul, my father, Charlotte, and Cheryl when we were visiting Vienna in 1972. The trip served as my family's first reunion with my parents following my departure from Hungary in 1956.

Figures 47-48. Left: The cottage at Badacsony, Hungary. Right: My Father is enjoying the view from the porch. The family cottage is located on the slopes of Badascony Mountain, where basalt rock once was excavated. Now excavations are against the law.

Figures 49-50. Pictured here are Dr. Bigelow (top) and (bottom) Drs. Heimbecker, Baird, Bigelow, and Key.

Figure 51. Just married! My lovely wife, Charlotte (maiden name: Scott), and I stand outside St. Clare Catholic Church in Toronto, Ontario, Canada, on our wedding day on June 27, 1964.

Figure 52. In 2010, Dr. Hanlon received the Lifetime Achievement Award of the American College of Surgeons (ACS).

Figure 53. Dr. Karl Klassen

Figure 54. A photograph of Glacier National Park that I took in July or August 1966.

Figure 55. Yellowstone National Park in the summer of 1966: bears and wild animals roamed freely in the park. In this photograph, a bear stands against a car window looking for some food.

PREFACE

᳁

My upbringing for many years was rather sheltered and highly protective. I was born and lived for twenty-five years in the separately standing Obstetrics and Gynecology Hospital of the Medical University of Pècs, Hungary. It provided great protection from the thunderous times of the 1930s and 1940s. I decided that I should reflect on them, since I can clearly remember most of the major events from early childhood. My family originated from Pècs but spread after World War II though Europe, North America, and the world. My brother is six years younger than me, and my sister is ten years younger. Both my siblings live in Hungary. My cousins and nephews live in different European countries: Sweden, Malta, Russia, Germany, and the UK. My own family lives in North America. Family exchanges will be difficult in the future, and nobody will be able to recall and understand the earlier stormy times of our family, unless I summarize them. During the years of upheaval during World War II, family members were too young to assimilate all that happened.

Fortunately, we all survived the war and the associated two brutal occupations of Hungary. Neither the German nor the Soviet regime tolerated individual rights, religious beliefs, or political differences. Escapes from concentration camps and political annihilations often occurred by serendipity. During the Holocaust, close to six million Jews were eliminated as well as millions more involved in other elements of resistance. According to estimates, Stalin killed twenty to twenty-five million people—nationals and enemies of the regime in the Gulag. The Nazi and Stalinist regimes annihilated basic human rights. Those people who resisted often were driven to death while trying to escape from behind the Iron Curtain or they joined the underground resistance, where they eventually got lost and disappeared.

During the Yalta conference, U. S. President Franklin D. Roosevelt sided with Stalin in the division of postwar Europe. The consequences of these unfortunate decisions were:

a) The people working for the Allies in the resistance movements of German-dominated countries, if not caught by the Gestapo, were turned over to the "Victors of the East." They were declared spies, fascists by the Soviets, and were deported to the Gulag.

b) Military units belonging to the East that were captured by Allied forces also were transferred to the Russians. The luckier, the younger ones, managed to survive and return to their countries. They lived through inhuman circumstances in different hard-labor camps in the Gulag.

The free-thinking people with revolutionary leanings always searched for a solution or an exit route. In 1956 the Hungarian Revolution against the occupying Soviet forces clearly reflected this situation. In 1956, two hundred thousand educated, mostly intelligent people left Hungary during the unexpected, three-month period of time, a "window," the only unusual opportunity in a fifty-year period during which the Iron Curtain was open. Hungary lost two percent of its most educated population; the individuals who fled the country never were allowed to return. For years, there was no chance for repatriation.

This was the time for "Carpe Diem." The defeat of the Revolution projected a most uncertain time period for future Soviet domination. It could have been decades or centuries. The West was engulfed in the dream of victory and did not realize the morbid consequences of Soviet expansion and the possible existence and spread of totalitarian regimes.

Reared under protective circumstances in relative isolation, I changed in response to the political situation and became a "revolutionary" escapee, looking for freedom, democracy, and better opportunities to achieve my professional dreams: an academic job, in which I would be able to perform what I always wanted to do—heart surgery. The opportunity was there; hard work paid off; I managed to have a lovely family and a relatively long and happy life.

This story of my life is what I call "An Incredible Journey."

PART I
THE FIRST TWENTY-FIVE YEARS:
OCTOBER 10, 1931- DECEMBER 14, 1956

THOMAS Z. LAJOS

HUNGARY UNDER NAZI INFLUENCE

MY FAMILY BACKGROUND

꧁꧂

MY FATHER'S FAMILY

My father's family was primarily one of teachers; my grandfather, Ferenc Lajos, was a principal; my great aunt also was a teacher. My grandfather's ancestors lived in Transylvania. My grandfather's father moved to Komarom, Hungary, where he was a shipbuilder.

The only relative I knew on my paternal grandfather's side was his sister, Ilus, the youngest of four children and three sisters. She married a lawyer and they lived in Tapolca, the neighboring city to Badacsony and the resorts of Lake Balaton in Hungary. For summer holidays, Ilus and her husband came to Badacsony, where they had a summer home, just like my other Grandaunt Erzsike (Elisabeth) Beke. Because Ilus's husband, Paul Csanyi, possessed "Hitlerian" leanings, we never had close relations with them, in spite of the fact that Badacsony was a very small, close community.

The Bekes, my paternal grandmother's family, originated from Northern Hungary. My paternal grandmother had a great number of relatives; for example, one of my great uncles had three wives and twenty-four children. I never could keep the Bekes straight in my mind. It seems I was not the only family member who found this difficult to do. While living in Buffalo, New York, I met a sales woman who was married to a Beke. She possessed only a vague knowledge of her husband's relatives but mentioned that her husband's relatives immigrated to the United States from Holland.

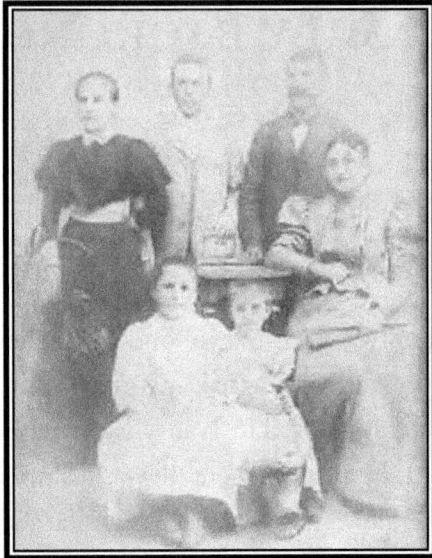

Figure 1. My grandfather, Ferenc Lajos, is standing to the right of his father in this photograph taken during the 1890s. My grandfather's three sisters also are shown. The youngest is my Great-Aunt Ilus, who sits in the front row.

I barely remember my Beke great grandmother, who died in the 1930s. My Beke Grandaunt, my grandmother's sister Erzsike (Elisabeth) Beke, was a school teacher. She lived with my paternal grandparents and never married.

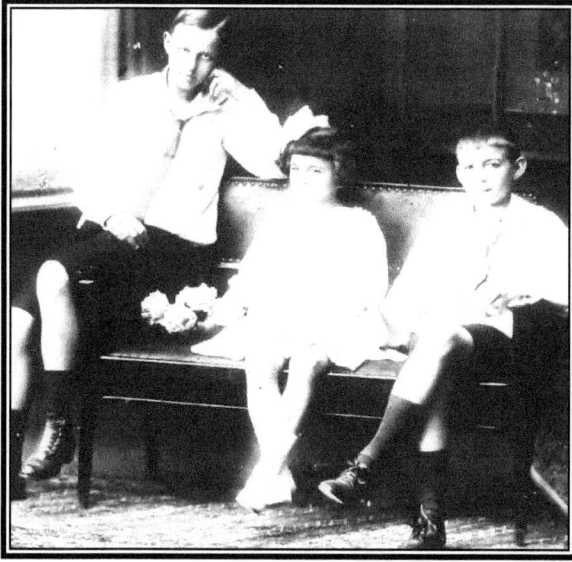

Figure 2. Taken in the early 1920s, this photograph shows my father, Laszlo, his sister, Jolan, and his brother, Ivan.

⌇

My father, Laszlo, was the oldest of my paternal grandparents' three children. My father's brother, Ivan, the middle child, was the most brilliant. My father's sister, Jolan, was the youngest. She eventually married Ferenc Newman, a gentleman of Jewish origin, and they moved to England before the Holocaust. They eloped and were married by one of our distant relatives, Reverend Laszlo Beke, a Franciscan priest, who lived in northern Hungary. My paternal grandmother and Great-Aunt Erzsike warned Jolan that if she married Ferenc Newman, she would not share in her inheritance of the cottage at Badacsony. The inheritance issue became the "Curse of Badacsony." My great-aunt had the cottage built adjacent to a small vineyard; Erzsike's total lifesavings was invested in that property. Jolan went to England and came back only to return permanently to the British Isles with her son, Ferike (little Ferenc). Ferenc (Feri) Newman's family owned a shoe factory in Szigetvar, Hungary. Feri pursued the same business later in Leicester, England.

After the Second World War, Feri and Jolan obviously wished to inherit the cottage in Badacsony with the rest of the family. The nationalization of private property under communist rule thwarted this hope. Furthermore, foreigners could not own private properties in Hungary. Only one way existed to keep the property in the family: one could save a second house or cottage from nationalization during the communist era, if it was dedicated to a prominent individual. The ownership of the cottage was transferred to my father, so the cottage was saved. This change in ownership eventually created a tremendous schism in the family. Many years after this initial family feud, it continued between my brother, my sister, and their families

MY MOTHER'S FAMILY

My mother's family, the Mantuanos, settled in Pècs during the early 1920s. The Mantuano family originated in Italy. The Mantuanos were traced to the crusaders, who liberated the Holy Land. The family was never rich, but diligent, hard-working, and middle class, if there was such a thing during those times (as noted by my relative Countess Judith Márffy-Mantuano Hare Listowel). At some time, the Mantuanos owned a chimney-sweeping firm in Nagykanizsa, Hungary.

My mother's father—my maternal grandfather, Jeno Mantuano, an engineer—started in Szeged, Hungary; then he moved his family to Pècs. He married Margit Fialovits from Nagykanizsa, the daughter of a furniture factory owner. The Fialovits' business went bankrupt during the Great Depression. Coincidentally, my wife Charlotte's maternal grandfather, an Armstrong, also owned a furniture factory that went bankrupt during the same Depression. The Armstrong factory was located in Guelph, Ontario, Canada.

Margit Mantuano, my maternal grandmother, gave birth to twin children: my mother, Julia, and her brother, my uncle Joseph. Joseph became an engineer like his father and eventually moved to Szekesfehervar and Budapest. My mother and my uncle were born on the same day in Szeged, and they amazingly died on the same day, ninety-four years later, while living apart in different cities! (my mother in Pècs and my uncle in Budapest). Does this prove twins truly are inseparable from each other throughout their lives and in death?

My grandfather Jeno's brother, Raoul, and Jeno's son Jozsef, my cousin, stunningly resembled each other.

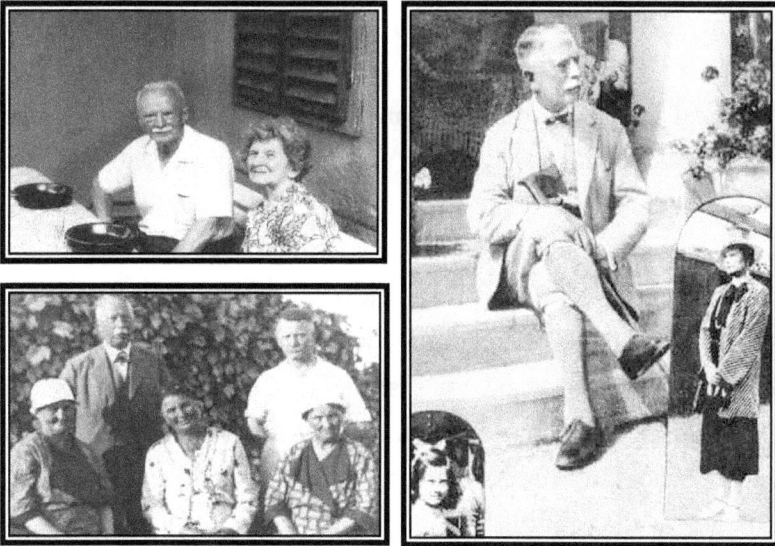

Figures 3-5. Top left: Twins, my mother and her brother, Joseph, are shown. Bottom left: Raoul, my maternal grandfather's brother, and Jeno, my maternal grandfather, respectively stand on the left and the right. They astonishingly resembled each other. Right: Mr. Raoul Marffy-Mantuano, my maternal grandfather's brother, sits in the sun on the doorstep of his Irmamajor mansion. Pictured respectively in the right and left insets are his wife and his daughter, Judith.

My maternal grandfather's brother, Rudolph (Raoul) Mantuano was a brilliant individual; he spoke six languages and was educated to be a diplomat. He became an attaché in Rome. He married into one of the "gentry families," the Marffys. Raoul did not invite his siblings to his wedding, a snub which created long-lasting family tensions. Raoul's daughter Judith became a reporter. She married the Fifth Earl of Listowel, William Hare, who was a communist and member of the postwar Attlee government. Supposedly, Lord Listowel's family denied him his inherited title. Judith and her husband eventually divorced; they had one daughter, Deirdre, who married Lord Grantley, who recently died. Deirdre remarried Mr. Ian Bayley Curteis, a playwright.

Deirdre's mother, Judith Listowel, wrote several books on family history as well as on Rudolf Habsburg's tragedy and the history of the Habsburg monarchy. Her book entitled *The Making of Tanganyika* described Tanzania and its first leader, Julius Nyerere. This book was well received. She claimed that David Livingston, the nineteenth-century Scottish missionary and explorer, never saw Victoria Falls in southern Africa; he only described it by means of hearsay.

Judith visited Hungary several times after the 1960s; my father and brother enjoyed her company on these occasions. My mother never forgave her, since Judith's father Raoul did not invite Jeno Mantuano, my maternal grandfather, to his wedding. Lady Listowel died recently at the age of 100.

My father and his brother Ivan were educated in the so-called "Realistic" School in Pècs. My paternal grandfather, Ferenc Lajos, was the principal at this school, which emphasized the sciences such as mathematics, physics, and chemistry, while the competing Cistercian-operated high school in Pècs emphasized art, music, literature, languages, and the humanities. Both my father Laszlo and Ivan were outstanding students; they successfully continued their studies at the University of Pècs, respectively studying medicine and law. My paternal grandparents anxiously provided the best educations for their children, even when they had to make financial sacrifices to do so.

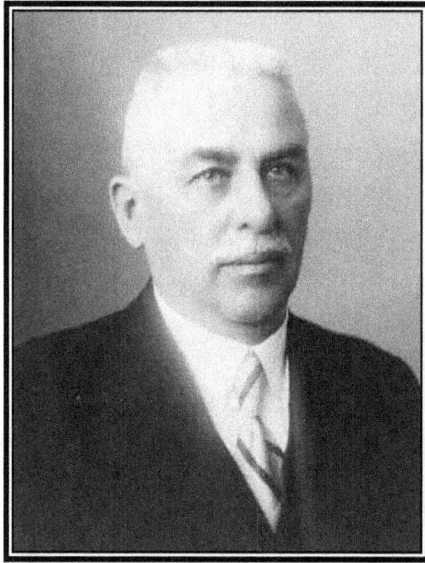

Figure 6. My paternal grandfather, Ferenc Lajos, Principal of the "Realistic School" in Pècs, Hungary.

When my parents married in 1928, my father was starting his clinical specialization in Obstetrics and Gynecology at the University of Pècs under the direction of a famous teacher and gynecologist, Professor Elemer Scipiades.

In 1931, when I was born, my parents lived within the confines of the main gynecology clinic building in a one-room apartment. Doctors were required to live in the hospital irrespective of the living conditions. By virtue of his ranking and status, the professor was given the best accommodations. He lived in a huge, multi-room flat that occupied half of the hospital's second floor wing. As my father progressed professionally, we moved to a roomier apartment; when he became the professor, we moved into the main building's wing.

The major depression started in the 1930s and lasted through the

1940s. Politically, the world was becoming more disturbed as Hitler's influence became more dominant in Europe. My father's good friend, Pista Peter, wanted my father and my mother to go with him on a vacation to Berlin, but my father refused; instead of using the money for a vacation, he bought himself a radio so he could listen to international broadcasting, the BBC and Radio Free Europe. Always working, he relaxed by listening to different broadcasts from the West until the Russian troops confiscated his radio after 1945.

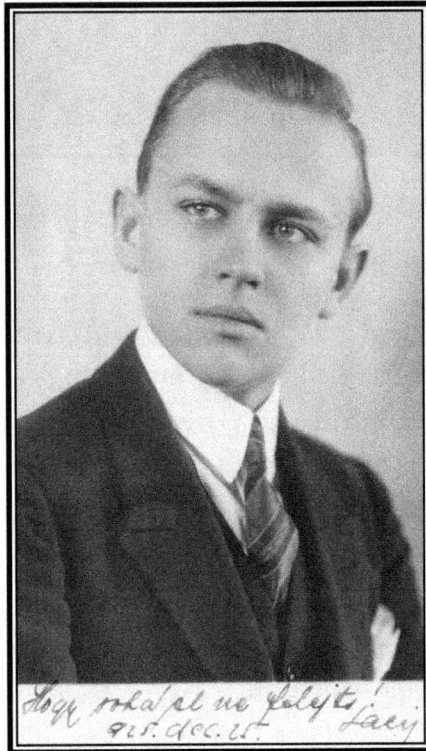

Figure 7. My father signed this photograph that he gave to my mother, "Don't ever forget me! Laci Dec. 25, 1925."

THE NAZI ERA IN HUNGARY

 ‿≈‿

My Uncle Ivan's book, *Germany's War Chances*, was published in 1939. Bound in Hungary with a rather simple, soft gray cover, it became known as the *"Szurke Konyv," The Gray Book*. It quickly became famous worldwide and rapidly was published in sixteen editions and six languages; thirty-six thousand copies were issued. The book's title concluded, *"Germany's War Chances: 'Germany Can't Win.'"* Under Nazi pressure, Hungarian officials took criminal action against its author.

My paternal grandparents lived on Rakoczi Ut for a long time before moving in later years to the apartments across from the University of Pècs. My Uncle Ivan was experiencing increasing political pressure after the publication of his book and was obliged to move to Budapest to be readily available to address repeated political and legal insults by the government and by Nazi-influenced public opinion. My grandparents followed to take care of him.

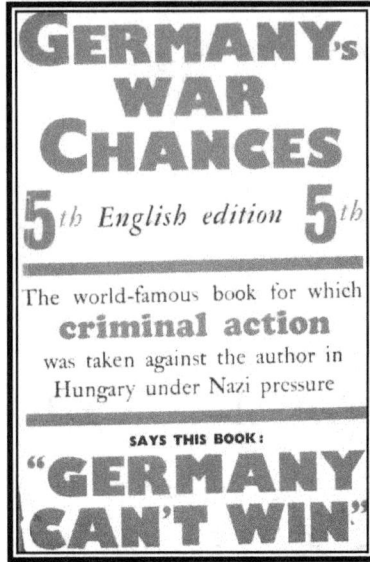

Figure 8. The front cover of the early English edition of my uncle Dr. Ivan Lajos's book.

We customarily visited Budapest for the Easter holidays. By now, my paternal grandparents had moved to Budapest from Pécs for convenience, because of my uncle's frequent commitments in Hungary's capital. My grandfather took us to the zoo on Good Thursday in 1941; I was ten years old, but I still clearly remember the family's despair that day upon returning home from the zoo to Raday Utca 30 felem.1. We found my grandmother and great aunt awfully upset and crying. My uncle had been taken to the Hadik, the military prison, for six days. I describe the circumstances of my uncle's imprisonment in my recently published book about Dr. Ivan Lajos's life, entitled *Fallen to Tyranny.*

My entire family's future and political stance were set from that time on, due to my uncle's anti-Nazi orientation during the Hitler era and anticommunist attitude during the Stalinist years. Ivan became engulfed in difficult legal and political situations. There was not any significant, organized left wing in the Parliament or underground resistance in the country; the 'legitimists' were the only opposition. Underground resistance cells operated practically independent from each other, with the exception of those supported by the British secret service. The public was poorly informed politically and was overrun by the political leaders, including Bela Gombos, Count Kalman Csaky, Bela Imredy, and Laszlo Bardossy. The Muscovite politicians were "recovering" and retrenching in Moscow following their defeat during the Spanish Civil War; they were preparing to seize power after the Second World War ended.

The Hungarian political leadership was aligning with Hitler's Germany, so the writing was on the wall: as my Uncle Ivan clearly foresaw in his book: "Hungary is going to side with the loser again for the second time in 30 years."

By participating with the Axis powers and declaring war against the Entente Powers, including the USSR and the United States, the "dice had been cast," thereby determining Hungary's political future, in spite of Admiral Horthy's lackluster efforts to extract the country from the war and its devastating outcomes. The seeds of more than thirty years of Hungary's political history were being planted when the country sided with the Germans and its allies.

Eventually my Uncle Ivan may have suffered a fate very similar to that of the famous Swedish diplomat Raoul Wallenberg, who arrived in Budapest in July 1944. Wallenberg's mission was to try to save some of the Jews being held in the ghettoes until they were deported for extermination.

Before the official Russian "liberation" of Hungary occurred on April 4, 1945, in January 1945, Wallenberg asked to see Russian General Malinowski in Debrecen, Hungary. Wallenberg never returned from this meeting; the Soviet secret service arrested him, accused him of spying, and imprisoned him in Moscow. Wallenberg's whereabouts in captivity and the circumstances of his eventual death in the prison or Gulag still remain unknown. The Russians have refused to shed a clear, definitive light on Wallenberg's fate. Similarly, my Uncle Ivan was taken by the Soviets, imprisoned, and convicted for crimes he never committed. The Soviets sentenced him to many years of hard labor in a Soviet camp in the Gulag, where he died. Our family never learned about Ivan's fate until it was too late.

MY FATHER'S PROFESSIONAL ADVANCEMENT AS AN ATTENDING PHYSICIAN AND ASSISTANT PROFESSOR OF OBSTETRICS AND GYNECOLOGY UNDER PROFESSOR ELEMER SCIPIADES

ี≥ผ

My father quickly progressed professionally. Professor Elemer Scipiades suffered a debilitating stroke in the early 1940s; he barely existed for two years. During this time, my father managed the entire OBGYN practice and clinic.

Professor Scipiades had been a stern, heavy individual, a dictator, a true "Geheimsrat." He directed the whole hospital and its administration with an iron hand. We were told as small children to greet him every time with a very loud "kezitcsoklom" ("I kiss your hand"), because he was hard of hearing. He often complained that he did not hear our greetings; yet when we raised our voices to greet him, he often complained that we were too loud and should not shout!

After Professor Scipiades died, my father relinquished to the Scipiades's family all the income that he had collected over the previous two years from the patients referred to the professor's practice. The Scipiades family graciously returned that money to my father. My parents used it to buy a drawing room furniture suite that was made by the best Hungarian furniture maker in Budapest. After the Russians seized Budapest, we thought that the furniture suite had been lost. My parents delightfully were wrong; the honest furniture maker disclosed that the furniture suite had survived in the part of the store that was not damaged. Remarkably every piece remained intact! My family still owns a few pieces of that furniture suite, which was shipped to America!

Professor Scipiades and his wife had three children—a son and two daughters. Elemer, the oldest, followed in his father's footsteps—he became a doctor and an OBGYN specialist. Nora, the elder daughter, married a doctor. About the same age as my mother, she was my mother's acquaintance and friend. Katinka, the youngest child, became a very talented musician, who studied piano in Budapest at the Hungarian Academy of Music. Katinka's husband, Erno Daniel, was a true musical genius—he became a pianist, conductor, and music teacher at a very young age. Erno played and gave piano concerts in Hungary and abroad. They had two children. After giving a piano concert in Rome, Erno did not return to Hungary; he defected, hoping to have Katinka and his children follow him. Erno's family was not permitted to leave the country; they unsuccessfully appealed to Mr. Hammarskjold, the Secretary-General of the United Nations. For at least ten years, Erno and his family lived separately and apart on different sides of the Iron Curtain.

After Professor Scipiades died, his family moved from Pècs to Budapest, where they owned a house. Katinka finally received an offer, a "kind of deal." She was permitted to leave Hungary with her two children in order to join her husband, if they surrendered their house with all its furniture, paintings, silver, rugs, and other valuables. Katinka accepted this "deal," to be reunited with her husband after twelve years of separation, in Santa Fe, New Mexico, U.S.A.. The Scipiades's house likely was taken by one of the high-ranking communist party members, who made the "deal."

Erno Daniel became a Professor of Music at the University of Southern California, Santa Barbara. After reuniting, the Daniel family lived together for only a few years. Shortly therafter, Erno Daniel died of leukemia at the age of fifty-six, having achieved a spectacular career as a pianist, conductor, and teacher. His elder son Erno Jr. became a cardiologist, living in Santa Barbara with a grown family. His sister Alexa married and became the mother of a nice family; she is a pharmacist, working in Salt Lake City. Alexa was a great support for her mother, who died in 2011 at 100 years old with very clear mind. Mrs. Daniel remained active until she died; she also was involved in music, teaching, and other activities. I received a handwritten letter from Mrs. Daniel around Christmas 2011, one week before she died.

My father possessed a firm, very decisive personality and required first-class performance from his associates as well as from us, his three children. If we brought home less than excellent school report cards, big family squabbles ensued, and we oftentimes were punished in different ways. We had to produce the best marks in school! I often thought my father went too far with these ideas. His rigorous attitude mellowed with my brother Laszlo the middle child, but he did not relax his high standards in my sister Judy's case. My brother probably was the smartest of the three of us.

In the early 1940s, when my brother "Lacko" was six years old, he started elementary school. Because he was extremely intelligent, he never had to work for good grades in school or the university. Consequently, he never learned to work hard, and work did not factor much into his philosophy of success.

My sister Judy was born in 1941; she is ten years younger than I am. She inherited all the good talents in the family: intelligence, diligence, and the resilience of the Lajos's. Even now, she is full of energy and only recently retired. Judy's daughter, Juditka, has a child, Niki. My sister's son Lacika lives in Germany with his two children, his daughter, Corina, and his son, Dominick (b. Nov. 2012).

While my father tried to "run" or manage his family with an "iron hand," sometimes his approach was not the most effective. My mother was an angelic soul, who followed my father's rules to a point while always managing to preserve her independence. After her gymnasium matriculation exam, she spent a year in Graz, Austria, to learn German, which she spoke, read, and wrote quite well. My mother's relationship with her in-laws was not always the smoothest and kindest, but she stood firm at times. Surely this created friction, sometimes fights, since my paternal grandmother always had to be right.

Somehow, I had a closer and sweeter relationship with my mother. She was not the most adept with money matters, and she certainly was not known for being the most punctual person. My father had to rule on these fronts: he allotted money for her daily activities and insisted that she be on time, in order to preserve his smooth professional and personal lives.

My mother loved to travel, and my father often said to her, "Iska, if you feel like traveling, I am happy to provide you with a first-class train ticket to Budapest and back." On one of these excursions outside of Pècs, I traveled with my mother to Prague to watch the Hungarian soccer team play against Czechoslovakia. (Incidentally, this pretext of going to support our country's soccer team was the only means whereby we could travel to another neighboring country during the late 1940s). We never saw the soccer game but thoroughly toured the city of Prague. What a beautiful city!

Early in the 1940s, my mother took me to the high Tatra Mountains for a couple of weeks to heal a possible "shadow" on my lung. I hiked everywhere and one day "climbed the Rysy." This peak provides the best view of the High and Low Tatras. In 1963, I managed to obtain a visa for my mother so that she could visit me in Toronto, Canada for the first time since I had left Hungary. Of course, I had to financially guarantee her entire trip and return to Hungary. When my mother was eighty years old, during the 1980s, she traveled with a group to Egypt to see the pyramids and other ancient sites there.

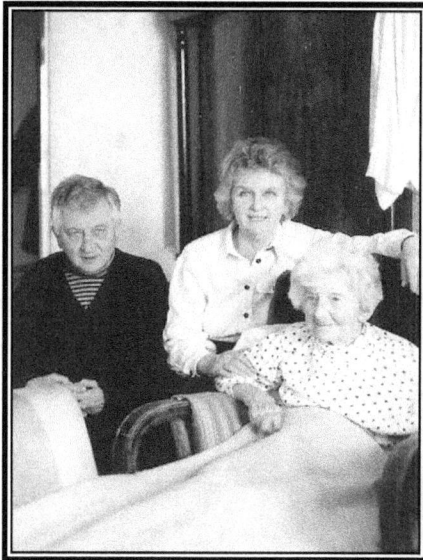

Figure 9. I took this photograph in March 1994 while visiting Pècs; my ninety-three year old mother is pictured here with my sister Judy (middle) and my brother Laszlo (far left).

As my father gradually advanced professionally, our family's lodgings improved too; we received a bigger apartment with more rooms and space. As members of the professor's family, we lived on the second floor of the main hospital building in the flat occupying about one-third of the second floor. A food elevator connected the kitchen on the ground level with the second floor. A woman who used to work for an aristocratic family cooked for us in the "kitchen." She was an excellent cook. In the European tradition, lunch was the biggest meal of the day, while supper was smaller. My parents had an ongoing social life with colleagues and friends.

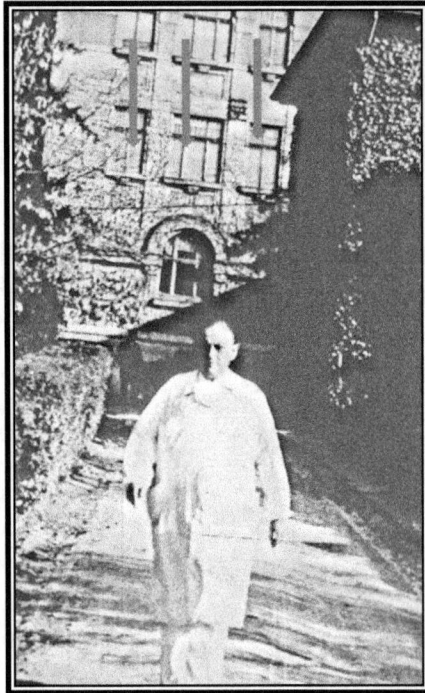

Figure 10. My father walks on the grounds of the Gynecology Hospital in Pècs. The arrows point to the three dining room windows of our flat on the second floor of the hospital.

My father did not speak foreign languages, but he appreciated, even later in his life, the necessity of learning them. He regularly took English lessons at home twice a week. Since the communist regime did not consider this type of learning acceptable, he studied languages at home behind closed doors. I too joined my father, studying English and French during private language lessons. While in high school I took French; during the 1940s, I took German in Maria Utca, Pècs, from a German lady, who probably was a Gestapo spy. Later at the University, where it was compulsory, I studied the Russian language; I never learnt it properly.

THE "SZULESZETI KLINIKA": THE OBSTETRICS AND GYNECOLOGY HOSPITAL

⌒⇋⌒

The Obstetrics and Gynecology Hospital, the Szuleszeti Klinika, was situated on a fifteen-acre fenced property with a rivulet running through the valley. Initially, this location encompassed a few freely-roaming deer, a swimming pool for the professor, and a tennis court for the doctors. A separate building housed the horses and eventually became a garage. Before motor vehicles were used, the horses transported food from the city of Pècs to the hospital.

The Medical University of Pècs's faculty occupied a Central Main Office building downtown. The different medical specialty clinics (Surgery, Internal Medicine, Gynecology and Obstetrics, Pediatrics, etc.) were scattered throughout the town. The various clinics or hospitals functioned independently: consequently, due to decentralization, services were cumbersome and expenses were high.

The garden at the Obstetrics and Gynecology Hospital was a splendid place; we roamed its fifteen acres while the deer grazed its grounds. We played with arrows and spears that we found there. We played tennis when the court was free. One day, my father had to pull me from a heavy snowdrift, in which I almost got lost. On another occasion, I pilfered and then ate a few strawberries that were growing in Professor Scipiades's garden. Its guardian reported me, and my father sternly punished me. "Those belong to the Professor!" When I exterminated a dirty alley cat from the garden, I received severe verbal lectures from the Nurses' Supervisor. Because the clinic was some two or three miles from the elementary school, I journeyed to and from school on a scooter. Surprisingly, nobody stole my scooter while it was parked in the school's entry hall.

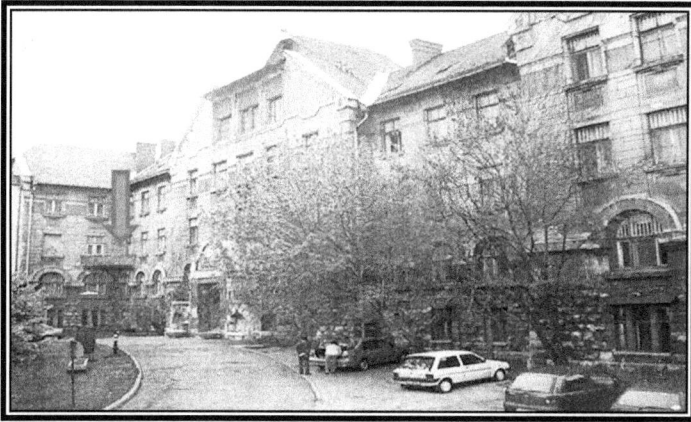

Figure 11. Another photograph of the Gynecology Hospital in Pècs. The arrow points to our apartment windows on the second floor.

The first floor of the Hospital Pavilion was the place we lived before we moved to the main building of the Hospital as my father advanced professionally. The hospital laboratory located on the top floor included a "dark room" for developing films. There I learned to develop my own films and photographs, and I experimented with different photo processes which existed at that time. Oftentimes we developed the films and paper with Zoltan Rozsnyai, an upcoming, young, talented conductor, who was a frequent visitor in Pècs. My acquaintance with Rozsnyai developed due to the fact that my father was planning to build an additional lecture theater adjacent to the main building. The designer's assistant for this project was Mr. Rozsnyai's wife.

Rozsnyai was one of the most talented young conductors in Hungary. He brought to Pècs many well-known artists, singers, violinists, pianists, orchestras, etc. during this period. Apparently after the 1956 revolution, he left the country too; he never became one of the leading conductors in the U.S.A.. He was notoriously late for his appointments! He conducted an orchestra once in Buffalo, New York, where I would live for many years, but afterwards, I did not hear too much about his activities and career. He may have died.

The lower floor of the Pavilion building housed the incurable cancer patients, often for palliative radiation as a last resort. Nitrogen Mustard was used as a chemotherapeutic agent, before Endoxan appeared in the 1970s. My father always used to say at that time, "The time will come when cancer patients have to be on chemotherapy for their lifetimes— just like those patients being treated for heart disease with digitalis." (My father's insightful vision of the future of cancer treatment was not far from today's reality.)

The living in the hospital compound was pleasant and well-protected. When it snowed enough, before the war got nasty, I often went to ski on Mecsek Mountain with the young doctors. At other times, we went "ski-joring." When there was not much traffic, the doctor who owned a car towed me at a reasonable speed behind his car while I was wearing my skis. This was a lot of fun! One day we came across a gypsy hut of very limited space in which the family was warming itself by a fire in the middle of the hut. The hut smelled, but the family received us in a friendly way. We had to watch our pockets during this visit.

My memories of World War II still are quite vivid. After the war started, one of the Jewish doctors was taken to the main German concentration camp Auschwitz and was exterminated. Another doctor, who was in the Hungarian army, fought at the River Don in Russia, where thousands of Hungarian soldiers were killed. When he returned, he stated that he would rather commit suicide than return to fight against the Russian army.

One day around noon while walking on the main Szechenyi square in Pècs, one of my classmate's parents told us that the Prime Minister of Hungary, Count Paul Teleky, had committed suicide on April 2, 1941. We could not understand how such a religious, practicing Roman Catholic could have taken his life. While all the circumstances surrounding Teleky's decision still remain unknown, we can surmise that he may have chosen to kill himself, because he could not face the fact that the Germans in Hitler's army had crossed Hungary's borders and were traversing towards the Balkans to fight against Yugoslavia. Teleky's recent peace agreement with the Allies was invalidated when the Germans crossed Hungary. He lost the opportunity with the U.S.A. and France to maintain Hungary's neutrality, curb the country's pro-Nazi orientation, and counter Hungary's drift to Germany's side.

Despite being only ten years old, I still remember well Prime Minister Count Teleky's tragedy. Probably this troubling incident was the first one that substantially impressed me or "shook my mind." One year later my Uncle Ivan's arrest and imprisonment in the Hadik, Hungary's military prison, was the next emotional trauma I suffered. From then on, the deteriorating conditions, the Hitlerian atmosphere, and the Russian occupation played a significant part in my decision to leave Hungary in 1956. My upbringing had been sheltered during these times until Ivan was deported to the German concentration camp Mauthausen and the Russians "liberated" Hungary. Hungary's complete loss of its sovereignty affected my political ideas and helped develop my ultimate decision to escape from behind the Iron Curtain.

Hungary was navigating "carefully" under the lack-luster rule of Admiral Horthy and slowly was overtaken by the Szalasi "Arrow Cross Party," which operated under totalitarian Nazi influence. By this time, the Hitlerjugend groups roamed and marched in the streets; they paraded in town and sang the Horst Wessel Lied ("The Flags Fly High") and other Nazi nationalistic songs.

Admiral Horthy was an admiral without sea! In his early years, he was an aide to the Kaiser Franz Joseph. Somehow he entered the marines and became a chief officer on a destroyer. He was victorious in one battle during World War I at Navarra on the Adriatic Sea. During the turmoil shortly after the end of the war and after the Treaty of Trianon (This peace treaty was signed in 1920 by the Allies and the Kingdom of Hungary in Versailles's Trianon Palace), Romania invaded Hungary. Horthy took the lead and kept the foreign troops out of Hungary. Riding on a white horse, he declared himself as the Regent and Governor of Hungary, established a military order for the loyal groups, and transferred to their members the title of "vitez" (This is the Hungarian word for "von" in German, meaning a lordship in English) by laying his sword on their shoulders. The title included some land and a farm. He vehemently objected to the restoration of a monarchy under the Habsburgs and prevented Karoly (Carl) IV's return to the Hungarian throne.

Horthy's army captured the king during his second attempt to return to Hungary and confined the king and his wife Zita to the Abbey of Tihany, at Lake Balaton. The king and queen stayed there until Horthy's army found the means whereby it could sentence Karoly IV and Zita to exile on Madeira and transport them there. When Karoly IV eventually died in 1922, he was buried on the island. En route to sainthood, he recently was beautified by the Pope. The Austrians made Karoly IV, King of Hungary, abdicate his throne; they confiscated his assets and land and forbade him to return to Austria. Incidentally, Karoly IV never used the word "abdication" in the document he signed. Bad Ischl Palace in Austria was left in the hands of the Habsburgs.

Karoly IV's wife Zita, a very energetic princess from Parma, Italy, died no more than ten years ago. Their son, Otto, a lawyer and member of the European Parliament, passed away at the age of 100 in 2011. My Uncle Ivan's book on Karoly IV was the first and probably the best biography ever written on his life.

THE GERMAN MILITARY OCCUPATION OF HUNGARY: MARCH 19, 1944

⸺⸺

Germany occupied Hungary on March 19, 1944, following a meeting between Admiral Horthy and Adolf Hitler. During this meeting between the two men—without interpreters present, since Horthy was fluent in German—a great brawl must have ensued. Horthy failed to extricate Hungary from the war—it probably was too late for this anyway—and in response, Hitler removed him from his Hungarian post and imprisoned the Horthy family in a Bavarian castle. In order to save his family, Horthy sacrificed Hungary and precipitated the German occupation.

On March 22, 1944, at midnight, there was a knock on my grandparents' apartment door in Budapest. The Gestapo deported my Uncle Ivan to the Mauthausen concentration camp in Austria with other Hungarian political prisoners.

When Mauthausen was liberated by the American troops on May 5, 1945, my Uncle Ivan was freed. In spite of his friends' advice (i.e. that of

Count Antal Sigray, George Pallavichini, George Parraghi, Horthy's son Miklos and others), Ivan returned to Hungary, the country he loved. Ivan and the other political prisoners were liberated just before they were to be executed like the other prisoners in Mauthausen. In the winter, naked outside in the freezing temperatures, prisoners were sprayed with cold water. Those who were still alive the next morning were shot by the Nazis.

While almost all of Ivan's friends from Mauthausen refused to return home to Hungary, Ivan returned to his homeland—Ivan's patriotism was unflagging. Promptly after returning to Hungary, he published two small booklets: *"Szotkerek" ("Let Me Speak Up")*, discussing and analyzing his predictions written before the war in the *"Szurke Konyv" (Germany's War Chances: 'Germany Can't Win')*, and *"The First Choice of Roads,"* analyzing Hungary's future. In preparation for the Paris Peace Conference scheduled for the fall of 1946, Ivan wrote the study, *"Magyarorszag felelosege a masodik Vilaghaboruban" ("Hungary's Responsibility in World War II")*, a copy of which he gave to Oxford University Professor Carlile Aylmer Macartney while they secretly met during the night at Ivan's apartment in February 1946. The Soviet regime in Hungary had tried to prevent Macartney from meeting with Ivan during his six-week visit to Hungary.

Given the political upheaval in Hungary, the Gynecology Hospital in Pècs surprisingly was unaffected. Politics were unknown within the hospital. Its doctors concentrated on delivering the best possible medical care to their patients. The pro-Nazi atmosphere in Hungary caused more anxiety. A few of the hospital's Jewish doctors were deported by the Germans. A Polish gynecologist, Dr. Bielewitz, had arrived a few years earlier. Nobody knew much about Dr. Bielewitz and why he had come to Hungary. I suspect my father was the only one who knew Dr. Bielewitz's true story. Dr. Bielewitz survived the German occupation of Hungary and left the country after the Russians ascended to power in 1946. He had been a prominent member of the Polish resistance.

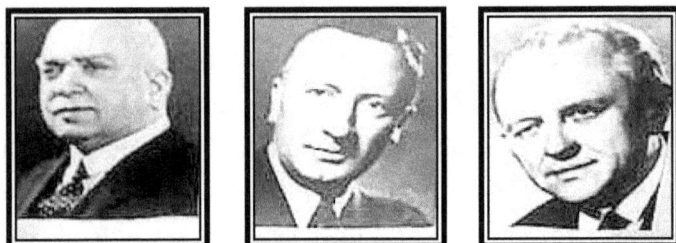

Figure 12. Professors Elemer Scipiades, Gabor Pal, and Laszlo Lajos are shown from left to right.

THE SOVIET INVASION AND OCCUPATION OF HUNGARY: APRIL 4, 1945

⌘

In 1944 the government appointed the outgoing Chief of Gynecology and Obstetrics from the University of Kolozsvar to the position of professor at the Gynecology Hospital in Pècs; he ranked over my father, who had been next in line. Dr. Gabor Pal was a hesitant, mediocre expert. He was Nazi-oriented and a poor Chief, who was afraid of the changing political scene. He wanted to move his family, the hospital, and the German troops westward to "escape" the Russian invasion. My father strongly objected and was determined to stay. The hospital staff stood behind my father and everybody stayed. Risking being shot or deported, my father led the procession outside in the snowy winter in front of all employees and doctors, when the Soviet troops entered onto the hospital grounds. Nobody got hurt or injured, except our mailman, who was killed by shrapnel a few days before. The hospital stayed open and was fully operational. By that time, the only resistance to the Russians was the German Wehrmacht.

Some of the clinic employees witnessed a remarkably horrific scene from the balcony of the Pavilion building. Watching the capitulation of a German soldier to the Soviet occupying forces, clinic employees saw the Soviets surround the soldier; they asked him to remove his boots and some of his clothing, even though it was in the middle of the winter and was snowy. The Soviet soldiers instantly appropriated the German soldier's belongings, and then they shot him in the back of his head, leaving him to die lying there in the cold. The Soviets used the same style of execution as they had during the revolution of 1918, during the time the Reds fought the White Russians on the Russian steppes.

During this time, I did "some business" and earned a few forints by selling cheaply obtained cigarettes at a higher price. The end to my entrepreneurial activities came when my father heard about them. He never was a good businessman.

For three months, under very rigorous and trying conditions, my grandparents withstood the siege of Budapest in their flat on Radai Utca. The corner room of the flat was penetrated by a cannon ball. All windows of the flat were broken. Food shortages ensued.

Pècs mostly escaped the ravages of Soviet sieges and their accompanying destructions. The battle at Pècs finished after a day or two, and damage was minimal. Atrocities, rapes, and killings were rare and/or nonexistent in Pècs, unlike in many other places in Hungary, like at the Abbey of Pannonhalma. There Bishop Vilmos Apor stood in front of the sections of the building in which the women were hiding, to protect the women from being raped by the Soviet soldiers. The Soviets killed the bishop on the spot.

American air raids continued, the war was still going on, and the group of "Liberators" (heavy bombers) flew sorties overhead—we thought to Ploesti, the Romanian oil-fields. They were performing "carpet bombings," which usually were executed in a rectangular or square fashion, totally destroying the designated areas. Frankfurt and Dresden were the primary victims with total destruction of both cities. Postcard pictures showed the damage caused by the carpet bombing of these cities. In Frankfurt, the cathedral was the only building left standing.

By now the Soviet army was reasonably well-equipped, thanks to material aid from the U.S.A. The "Stalin organ" and Soviet tanks were the dreaded weapons. By means of the "Stalin organ," the Soviets used multiple cannons grouped together to deliver destructive fire to a designated square or rectangular area. Usually nothing remained where the bombs hit!

(Incidentally, the Libyan rebels were well-supplied with these old-fashioned Russian cannons when they fought Muammar Gaddafi. We saw them on television during the Libyan affair.)

A couple of the U.S. bombers—"Liberators" as they were called—performed an emergency landing in the small airport at Pècs. They never bombed us in Pècs. The airmen supposedly were picked up by the Soviets and deposited in the best hotel, the Nador, until they returned to their units. The war raged during these times in Budapest (for three months) and in Berlin. The American pilots were very friendly individuals; they talked freely to us, gave us chewing gum, which we did not have at that time, and showed us their high caliber hand guns, Colts that hung on their belts. Stupidly, I engaged in a discussion about guns with them and mentioned that I owned a BB air handgun. One of the soldiers asked me to show it to him, since he had not seen one. When he looked at it the next day, he liked it so much that he took it!

Rebuilding after the occupation was difficult. People had lost their houses and relatives; there were food shortages; inflation set in, the highest ever recorded in *The Guinness Book of World Records*. Organization was nonexistent. As "true occupiers," the Soviets and their troops ransacked the country, raping women and girls, shooting some clergymen, stealing household utensils, and collecting all weapons and radios.

When the Soviets entered my maternal grandparents' flat in Pècs, at Maria Utca 17.sz, they intended to empty it. They stabbed a bayonet into the well-made beds to be sure that people were not hiding under the covers. The female soldier assigned to live in their flat bitterly complained that because the water was running too fast from the toilet, she had no time to wash her face. This soldier took a pail of water outside in the middle of the winter to wash herself. Soviet soldiers took peoples' wrist watches from their wrists when they noticed them, saying "davai chasi" ("Give me your watch"). Forty years later, when Soviet troops withdrew from Hungary, they similarly conducted themselves; they looted from their specially-built quarters; they took home the bathroom taps, toilet bowls, sinks, and piping, among other things of value.

AT TELEP ON LAKE BALATON

❧

My schooling was interrupted periodically during the war. In 1943 and 1944, the beginning of each school year was delayed by two months. I spent those most pleasant and happy months—September and some of October—with my maternal grandparents in Telep at their estate on the southern shore of Lake Balaton. They owned three to four acres of land, partially grapevines and trees, on the lake shore. Somehow I managed to take care of my Uncle Joseph Mantuano's rented sailboat, which I used almost every day whenever possible. Before I departed every morning on the sailboat, my grandmother told me to be careful and to be back for dinner on time—and I was. My maternal grandparents were exceptionally understanding, nice, and peaceful people. They were the best grandparents any grandson could have. Happiness and love were in the air at their home at all times! I spent my happiest summers with my maternal grandparents at their estate in Telep.

I took sailing trips often during the summers of the late 1940s, with the most awful, old sailboats, but I was exceptionally happy when we managed to secure a class boat like the "Pirot." I sailed to Keszthely from Maria and Gyorok and to Balatonfüred, which was located in the north basin of the lake. The narrowest part of the lake is at the tip of the Peninsula of Tihany and Szántód, on the south shore. There the lake narrows to less than a mile across. Lake Balaton is the deepest at its narrowest juncture, about ten meters deep. The narrowest part divides the lake into two basins: the North and the South. As a result of cross currents, the narrowest part became the deepest.

Some of my sailing trips lasted for a couple of days, during which I camped without a tent upon the shore. One day, my brother and I decided to sail across the lake from Telep to Badacsony (fifteen to twenty kilometers) to see my paternal grandparents on the north shore for a short time. In the afternoon, we decided to return to Telep. There was a brisk north wind, which made running with an oversized mainsail quite tricky. Sure enough, three to four kilometers out in the lake, off the shadow of the southern facing Badacsony mountain—the remnant of a volcanic eruption of basalt stone, providing an ideal climate for superior wine production—we capsized, while wildly running downwind to the south. My grandfather witnessed this event from the shore. Luckily, the ferry from the southern port of Fonyód had just passed us; it turned around, rescued us from the water, and towed our boat to the shore. We stayed overnight in Badacsony and returned to the south shore the next morning after completing minor repairs on the boat. For a long time, we did not dare to admit this incident to my father.

Telep
Balaton - Máriaalsó

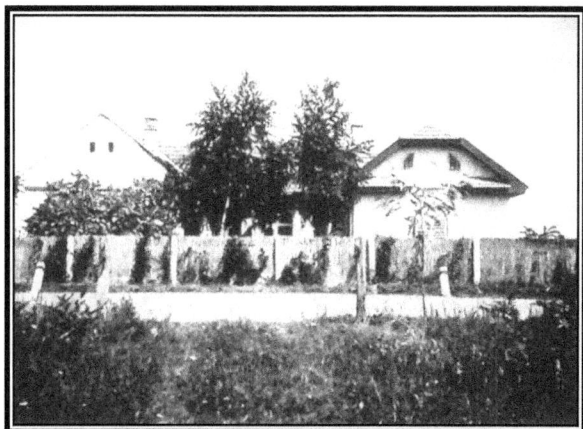

Figures 13-14. Top: my maternal grandparents' family cottage at Telep. Bottom: At Telep on Lake Balaton in 1943, my maternal grandparents go for a walk.

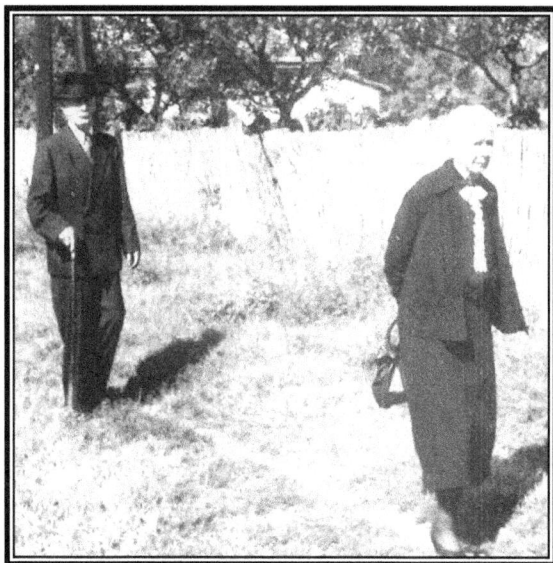

LAKE BALATON: THE SECOND BIGGEST LAKE IN EUROPE

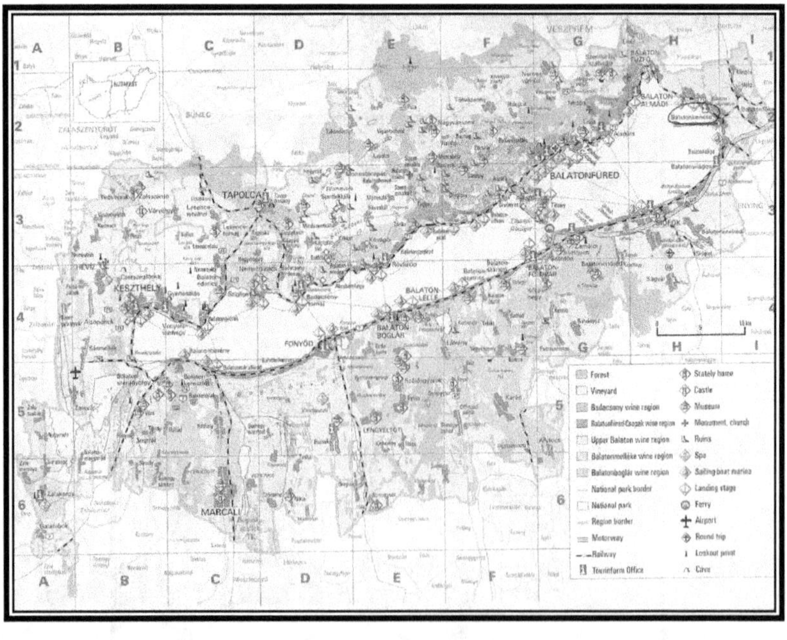

Figure 15. Lake Balaton is the second biggest lake in Europe. The line (D4) between Fonyód (on the south shore) and Badacsony (on the north shore) indicates the ferry route.

On the north shore at Badacsony, where the cottage belonging to my paternal grandparents and grandaunt was located, we often had tense moments within the family, which at times were not fully understood. In retrospect, I can see some of the reasons for the tensions and strained relations: my aunt was in England, absent for years by now, and my uncle was in the Nazi concentration camp Mauthausen.

One year after my Uncle Ivan returned, he disappeared from Budapest in June 1946. We never knew anything about his fate for over fifty years. These circumstances undoubtedly were almost unbearable for my paternal grandmother. She was the matriarch of the family, who fought for her family, defended its members, and guided them throughout hard times. In later years, my paternal grandmother never accepted that my Uncle Ivan would not come home; she did not know that he had been taken to the Gulag, where he died.

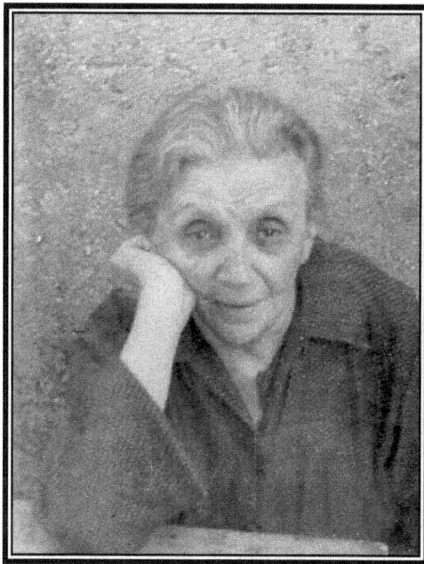

Figure 16. A photograph of my paternal grandmother taken in the early 1960s.

The dining room table in Badacsony had a heavy round base that was utilized to hide my uncle's writings and other relics remaining after the Soviets raided my grandparents' flat in Pècs. My grandparents' home first was ransacked by the Nazis in 1939 and later by the Russian Secret Police in 1946, when they invaded Hungary under the pretext of "liberating" it. A copy of my uncle's personal diary was given to my grandfather, who hid it in the table, but it eventually was lost. The other copy of Ivan's diary was handed to a member of the British Legation, who was stationed in Budapest in 1946, one month before Ivan disappeared. To my knowledge, this copy of Ivan's diary was given to Mr. Frank Gann Redward.

Mr. Redward's papers are preserved in the British Archives at Kew, where they will not be unsealed before 2031. While a copy of my Uncle Ivan's diary is believed to exist, perhaps in Mr. Redward's papers, its whereabouts remains an unsolved mystery for our family. If discovered, it likely will reveal a tremendous amount of information about the political situation in Hungary during and then shortly after World War II when the Soviets began to rule in Hungary.

My grandfather and father often went fishing together; they enjoyed nature, the lake, and its sunsets and sunrises. Camaraderie existed among the fishing gentlemen in Badacsony. On one of these fishing trips, my grandfather and father befriended József Egry (b. 1883- d. 1951), one of the greatest Hungarian painters of the twentieth century.

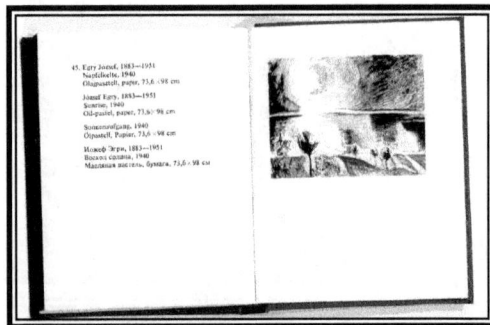

Figure 17. Mr. József Egry. The Lights of Lake Balaton.

Our cottage in Badacsony became the yearly summer excursion place for many of my father's colleagues and friends. In one of those years, József Egry offered to show his paintings, in his art studio on the top of his four-story, four-room (i.e. each floor had one room) house, located on the harbor with a lake view. Egry extended his personal invitation to show his paintings to my father, his friends, and me. Egry stacked his paintings in his studio, where, during the showing, he pulled the most beautiful canvases from his stacks. Most of the works we saw were representations of the "play" of lights on Lake Balaton. The artist was friendly and optimistic; he did not show any signs of his chronic depression during our visit. He had tuberculosis that finally killed him.

The richness and beauty of Egry's art works were amazing. Nowadays because they are national treasures and extremely expensive, if one wants to buy one of Egry's paintings, one has to obtain the permission of the Hungarian government and pay thousands of dollars for each masterpiece, including high taxes. The authorities usually do not give permission to remove any of Egry's works from the country. They are now considered cultural property of Hungary.

MY HIGH SCHOOL "GYMNASIUM" YEARS: 1942-1950

I n 1942, my father decided to enroll me in the school operated by the Cistercians, rather than in the one run by the Jesuits; he argued that the Cistercians were more down-to-earth. There was great rivalry between these two schools in Pècs.

The Cistercian order of priests uneventfully ran my high school, the Nagy Lajos Gymnasium, until the political situation started to change in Hungary. The school was liberal and humane. Even during the Nazi regime in Hungary, Jewish students did not have to wear the yellow Star of David inside the school. After the "Soviet liberation" of Hungary, the Soviets increasingly pressured the priest-teachers until the communists deported them to labor camps in 1948.

At the beginning of the twentieth century, Mór (Maurice) Kármán developed the Hungarian education system in conjunction with the Austro-Hungarian education system. It was nurtured by Franz Joseph I (b. 1830-d. 1916), the Emperor of Austria and the King of Hungary.

Children started four years of elementary school when they were six-years-old, and continued their educations through higher schools or universities. Successful graduation from higher schools, called "gymnasiums," which were roughly equivalent to American middle and high schools, took place after eight years of study. Gymnasium education could be more oriented to and based upon either the sciences—such as chemistry, mathematics, physics, and biology—or the humanities including literature, languages, music, arts, etc. Graduation came after one completed the "biggest examination," the matriculation, the final gymnasium graduation and exit exam, written in one day, followed by a one-day oral examination. One either made it by passing the examination or one had to repeat the last year! Certain high schools had early specialization, like the Minta School, the gymnasium of languages, and the high school in Godollo specializing in French.

Mor Kármán, the founder of the celebrated Minta School, was an educator of Jewish descent rather than a wealthy businessman. The Hungarian Jewish middle class produced seven exceptional scientists, all from Northern Hungary and educated on the same educational principles professed by Kármán. Without exception, these men were driven hard by their parents and by the social circumstances. Listed here in the order of their births, they were the son of Mor Kármán, Theodore von Kármán (b. 1881-d. 1963), George de Hevessy (b. 1885- d. 1966), Michael Polanyi (b. 1891- d. 1976), Leo Szilárd (b.1898 – d. 1964), Eugene Wigner (b. 1902– d. 1995), John von Neumann (b.1903 – d. 1957), and Edward Teller (b. 1908– d. 2003). These men, most of them earning the Nobel prize, made major contributions to science and technology.

Edward Teller and Leo Szilárd were graduates of the Minta School. Teller and von Neumann became close friends. One time years later, when the group discussed the development of the atomic bomb, one of them said: "We could talk Hungarian." The only non-Hungarian speaking scientist who developed the atomic bomb was Enrico Fermi from Italy.

Basic sciences were taught in the first two years of the university. At U.S. colleges, these basic science courses serve as preparation for upper level undergraduate courses in the science majors. In Hungary, in preparation for the medical degree, the first two years of university studies concentrate on the basic sciences, including mathematics, physics, chemistry, and biochemistry. The last two years of medical education at the university level were spent on the clinical specialties (i.e. medicine, surgery, gynecology, obstetrics, neurology, forensic medicine, etc.). University education in medicine was followed by a year of studying each of the clinical specialties for three months. Graduation ensued after full university training in medicine.

The so called "college years," as they are known in the U.S., were absent in Hungary. They were unnecessary and would have been superfluous, because at the age of eighteen, following the matriculation exam, university entrants were nearly sure what professions they wanted to practice in the future. In the "realistic" gymnasiums they began studying basic sciences in the final years: mathematics, geography, chemistry, physics, geology, etc.

In my opinion, in general, a school and its teachers may be excellent, good, and/or mediocre. Without a doubt, the educators at my high school—the priests—were extremely dedicated. Teaching was their vocation, besides the priesthood!

Father Allan Eber, the religion teacher, was a genius; he organized concerts, operas, and plays and built a swimming pool. Later he was found dead in a boat floating on Lake Balaton. Eber's cause of death was not determined; he may have committed suicide or died suddenly. Father Akos Kelecsenyi continuously badgered us: "You are educated on 'sports newspapers.'" He eventually left the priesthood, quit his order, and probably married. My main teacher and the principal of my class was Father Roman Felegyi, a simple, straightforward, good individual. I visited him during my first return visit to Hungary. At his home, he was taking care of his sick mother, who had suffered a debilitating stroke.

While they may have been religious and devoted to God, some of these teachers often were impossible; some possessed uncontrollable tempers, like those of madmen: Dezso Modly, Szaniszlo Kuhn, and Mr. Shiptar, the German teacher. One thing was true—they did not discriminate against anybody, not even against Jewish students or the gypsies.

Some of my teachers could be rather incriminating as they tried to convert students to the priesthood. Two of my classmates became priests. The first classmate, Father George Timar, recently died from natural causes. My other classmate, Father Janos Brenner, will become a saint. He is a "modern" Saint Tarsicius. One night during the communist era, while carrying the Eucharistic host to a dying individual, he was stabbed to death in his village by a group of gangsters, who never were apprehended or brought to justice. The identities of Father Brenner's assailants still remain unknown. Witnesses were non-existent or unwilling to come forward. Consequently, the circumstances of his death remain shrouded in mystery.

One of the "star" Cistercian priests, Father Bernardin Pallos, was a German sympathizer and unlike his prominent order-mate, Father Justine Baranyai, a staunch legitimist and friend of my Uncle Ivan. Baranyai became involved in the Cardinal Jozsef Mindszenty trial and was sentenced to fifteen years in prison. Father Balduin Opperman was a highly respected Latin teacher; Father Miksa Gombas, of literature, and Father Adolf Horvath, of botany. In later years, Horvath received the Kossuth prize for botany. Father Gothard Kertesz taught geography. Horvath and Kertesz were the most outstanding teachers, held in the highest regards by students. I met Father Vendel Endrédy, Abbot and head of the Hungarian Cistercians in Zirc Monastery. He knew of my Uncle Ivan. As I learned recently, Endrédy was tortured later on and physically weakened. The students' mothers favored Fathers Ipoly Nyolcas, Jacinth Barna, and Oliver Santha.

Around 1947-8, the Cistercian teachers were deported overnight to labor camps; civilian teachers assumed the responsibilities of providing our educations. During the last two years of my eight years of gymnasium, I was taught by non-priest teachers.

Mr. Mihály Temesi was the only civilian teacher I respected and liked. A highly intelligent individual and a linguist, he served as the French teacher. He had become a teacher and a professor in the Postgraduate Teachers College, Pécs. His basic science studies pertained to the development of the Hungarian language. He used to philosophize while teaching about materialism and religious beliefs. He tried to "sharpen" and "broaden" the students' ideas beyond the dialectic materialism, as taught by the Communist Party. Recently, he was accused of being a communist, but the government rehabilitated him. I was asked to write a short testimony about his outstanding teachings and character. The other civilian teachers I would rate as average.

The matriculation exam was offered at the end of the eighth year of the high school gymnasium. At that time, in 1950, I had to choose a profession. Under the dictatorial system, there were few sane career choices; they consisted of careers in the sciences, medicine, or one of the engineering specialties. My interests in the humanities—including history, international law, and diplomacy—would not have sustained a viable and fruitful career under that Hungarian regime. For my future career, I envisioned but one and that was medicine, the only choice remaining from the few offered.

I had to take a university admission examination in spite of my excellent high school grades. I was a child of parents who belonged to the "intelligentsia," so I was required to take it in order to gain entrance to the university. The regime established a university admissions quota for the children of intelligentsia. Unlike for peasants' and laborers' children, only a restricted number of children from the intelligentsia were admitted to the universities. They had to score highly on the matriculation and university admission exams. Admitted to the universities without having to take the entrance exams, sons and daughters of the favored labor class and small landowner peasants enjoyed the privileges of the regime! Was this the same as "numerus clausus" during the 1920s, which was used to exclude individuals of Jewish descent from studying at the universities? My brother and his wife, both of whom studied law at the university level, were excluded similarly from practicing law in Hungary. They endured tough times because of these political policies.

THOMAS Z. LAJOS

THE IRON CURTAIN

"SALAMI" POLITICS IN HUNGARY

⌒≋⌒

D uring my early high school years in the Nagy Lajos Gymnasium, the Cistercians operated the school undisturbed by the government or its policies. However, in 1948 the political situation in Hungary started to change; my school was greatly affected.

The dominant political party, the Kisgazda (i.e. Little Land Owners Party) ruled the country by democratic elections with a majority vote, but it still had to share important cabinet posts with the communists. The Chief of the Communist Party, the Moscovite Mátyás Rakosi, served as the Co-Prime Minister of Hungary. In addition, the Secretary of Internal Affairs also was a communist—Mr. László Rajk, who was eventually executed by Rakosi due to unresolved rivalry.

Hungary was at this point a parliamentary democracy with one house, a President, and a democratically-elected government. The leaders of the democratic parties served as politicians for years during the Horthy era, but certainly lacked the shrewd manipulative powers of the communists. Most of the communist Muscovites were trained in Moscow and participated in a short-lived Hungarian communist regime with the

Hungarian communist leader Béla Kun, who also was executed during the 1930s in Moscow.

Some of these communist leaders also participated in the Spanish Civil War later. These communist leaders, one by one, infiltrated the Democratic Party. By 1948, during repeated elections, the communists established one list of candidates and then obtained a ninety-eight percent majority, without opposition. The existing Prime Minister, Ferenc Nagy, fled to Switzerland to save himself and his family.

Incidentally, my father had operated on Mrs. Nagy a few years before and afterwards received as a small gift, a good-sized (14" x 16" inches), autographed photograph of the prime minister. The authorities a few years later found this picture sitting on the top of my father's office bookcase. It caused a lot of trouble, and my father was required to "explain" it.

Several times, the prime minister and his family were guests at my parents' home, but due to the political situation in Hungary, Nagy was more or less a sitting duck politically and was powerless. When my Uncle Ivan disappeared in 1946, even Nagy was unable to use his ties to locate Ivan or determine that he was being held, accused of political crimes. Ivan had been imprisoned in the Soviet's Control Committee building in Budapest.

Working as a part of the Inter-Allied Control Committee in Budapest for three months, the Soviet's Control Committee was free to operate; the western powers did not interfere with its affairs. In fact, the western powers (i.e. the Americans, British, and French) left Hungary entirely in the control of the Soviets. This hands-off approach of the western powers was summarized by the following terms: "What is in the East, it belongs to the East; it belongs to the Soviet authorities!"

During these uncertain times, the communists dissolved and then in some cases re-formed the radio stations, news media, publishing companies, and other youth, social, and political organizations. Social organizations, including artistic and religious groups, were eliminated initially by infiltration and attrition and later by "higher orders."

In December 1945, a Russian colonel and an unknown woman by the name of Natasha visited my Uncle Ivan in his Budapest flat in Raday Utca 30.1/2 em.#1. They asked Ivan to have discussions with them at the Soviet Control Committee's building. On June 17, 1946, my Uncle Ivan left his home and never returned again. For fifty-two years, until January 6, 1998, nobody in our family knew Ivan's whereabouts or what happened to him. Only in response to my brother's repeated inquiries, in 1998, the Soviet and Hungarian governments issued Ivan's "rehabilitation papers" to our family, revealing that he died on September 10, 1949, from tuberculosis and emphysema while imprisoned in one of Stalin's work camps in Tartoul, Kazakstan, Karaganda. I describe my uncle's fate in considerable detail in my book *Fallen to Tyranny*.

As Hungary was a Soviet "occupied country" and member of the Warsaw Pact, its borders were sealed by automatic guns, machine guns, mines, and barbed wires, all of which operated on a synchronized alarm system. Its neighboring countries also were included in the strict travel restrictions.

The western border of Eastern Europe had been sealed by the Iron Curtain as Winston Churchill described it in his Iron Curtain Speech, delivered at Westminster College in Fulton, Missouri on March 5, 1946:

From Stettin in the Baltic to Trieste in the Adriatic an iron curtain has descended across the Continent. Behind that line lie all the capitals of ancient states of Central and Eastern Europe: Warsaw, Berlin, Prague, Vienna, Budapest, Belgrade, Bucharest and Sofia. All these famous cities and the populations around them lie in what I must call the Soviet sphere, and all are subject, in one form or another, not only to Soviet influence but to a very high and in some cases increasing measure of control from Moscow.

The sharp division between east and west occurred because of the unfortunate failure of American foreign policy at Yalta in the Crimea in 1945. Franklin D. Roosevelt was seriously ill at the time. He had a metastatic brain tumor caused by malignant melanoma. Unfortunately, he sided with Stalin, when sound decision-making was paramount. The absence of good decision-making at Yalta was similar to the situation after the World War I, when U. S. President Woodrow Wilson and his Secretary Secretary of State were overruled by French statesman Georges Clemenceau. The two Czechoslovakian politicians, Edvard Benes and Tomás Masaryk, exerted significant influence. Middle Europe, specifically the Austro-Hungarian territories, were dismantled by the Versailles Peace Treaty. The size of Hungary was significantly reduced; territories were assigned to the surrounding nations (ex. Erdely to Romania, northern Hungary to Czechoslovakia and southern Hungary to Yugoslavia), without regard for minority ethnic groups, including substantial Hungarian populations living within them. Germany and its allies also bore the unbearable repercussions of the Versailles sanctions.

President Woodrow Wilson had only a few good ideas about how to preserve the balance of power in Europe, and his secretary of state suffered from the same shortsightedness! Borders were reconfigured erratically without consideration of ethnic and geographical factors. Ethnic groups found themselves on the "other side" of well-established national borders that had existed for centuries. The geographies of national resources were ignored. Families were divided by the new borders. Ethnicity did not count! Ethnic cleansing was the rule of the victors! Unquestionably, this type of ethnic discrimination continued after World War II, pioneered by the Soviets!

At the end of World War II, the Yalta agreement dictated that U.S. troops had to stop at the Elbe River. The East was to be occupied by the late-arriving Soviet troops and remained in Soviet hands for decades.

U. S. Army General George Patton's fierce objection to stopping at the Elbe was overruled. Berlin was given to the Soviets, resulting in its complete isolation. Berlin was surrounded and blockaded. A single road connected West Berlin to the West. As part of the Marshall Plan (officially the European Recovery Plan, ERP), the U.S. had to establish airlifts to West Berlin in order to provide the divided city with supplies, food, and other assistance. Only Winston Churchill and a few others countered Stalin's expansion policies.

Hungary became overburdened with war reparations owing to the USSR and Czechoslovakia. It was ordered to respectively pay $200 million and $100 million in war damages. The borders of the country were reduced again to those set forth in the Versailles Treaty after World War I. The country and its peoples were thrown to the Soviets! Millions of ethnic Hungarians in Slovakia, Yugoslavia, and Romania also suffered discrimination!

Only Communist Party members and a few internationally renowned scientists and musicians were able to travel to the West, due to imposed travel restrictions. Travel between the Warsaw Pact nations also was difficult for most individuals. Money transfers and exchanges were limited while trade with the West became non-existent. Complete political and economic isolation ensued. If Hungarians corresponded with people in the western nations, their actions caught the attention of communist authorities. These Hungarians were lucky to avoid arrest; their activities were recorded in secret police dossiers maintained by the Hungarian Secret Police, the AVO. In her book, titled *The Enemies of the People*, Katie Martin discusses in great detail how the communist takeover of Hungary affected educated and cosmopolitan Hungarians such as her parents, who were imprisoned for their activities involving foreign correspondences and contacts.

Throughout the Hungarian cities, the communists established "town hall" meetings to popularize the communist doctrine of dialectic materialism. Initially, at the beginning of the transformation of the regime, democratic debates occurred and were allowed. These meetings were interesting and fascinating, particularly when philosophers and/or Jesuits participated as opponents. By well-reasoned, sound arguments, the Jesuits, without any doubts were most of the time victorious. They debated and defeated Communist Party members, who represented the tenets of dialectic materialism. Realizing they were not winning these town hall sessions, and thereby not convincing the people, the communists discontinued these discussions. They eventually eliminated all oppositional, "social" associations, groups, and organizations, as the beginning of "Stalinization." (The expression of "The Stalinist Homo" was coined by Anne Applebaum in her book *The Iron Curtain*; it refers to individuals who became Stalinized).

Under the new communist regime in Hungary, the party members were obliged to address each other, even in Hungarian, as "Comrade" Green or "Comrade" Weiss, for instance, and not as Mr. Green or Mr. Weiss! Not surprisingly, the word "Comrade" in the Hungarian language is nonexistent. The Hungarian Party members called each other "Elvtars." That word consists of two words combined: "Elv" meaning "principle" and "tars" meaning "my fellow." Those communists certainly were not my "fellows" and friends in "principle."

THE "IRON CURTAIN" DESCENDED FROM NORWAY TO THE MEDITERRANEAN: 1946

⟿

The Iron Curtain isolated the East from the West, from Kirkenes, Norway, to the Mediterranean Sea. The Berlin Wall divided Berlin into East and West Berlin and put Berlin itself into the Soviet zone. One corridor of land—a road—connected Western Europe with West Berlin. The Berlin Wall became the symbol of the division between the East and West during the Cold War. This was "the road to death" if one chose to cross it.

Obstacles, mines, barbed wire, high fences, and watchtowers with guards and automatic guns were built and operated in order to keep people within the Soviet block and prevent illegal immigration to the West. Photographs and blueprints reveal the ten layers of border reinforcements. The "arms of the devil" clearly were built into this system, making it nearly impossible for individuals to escape to the West.

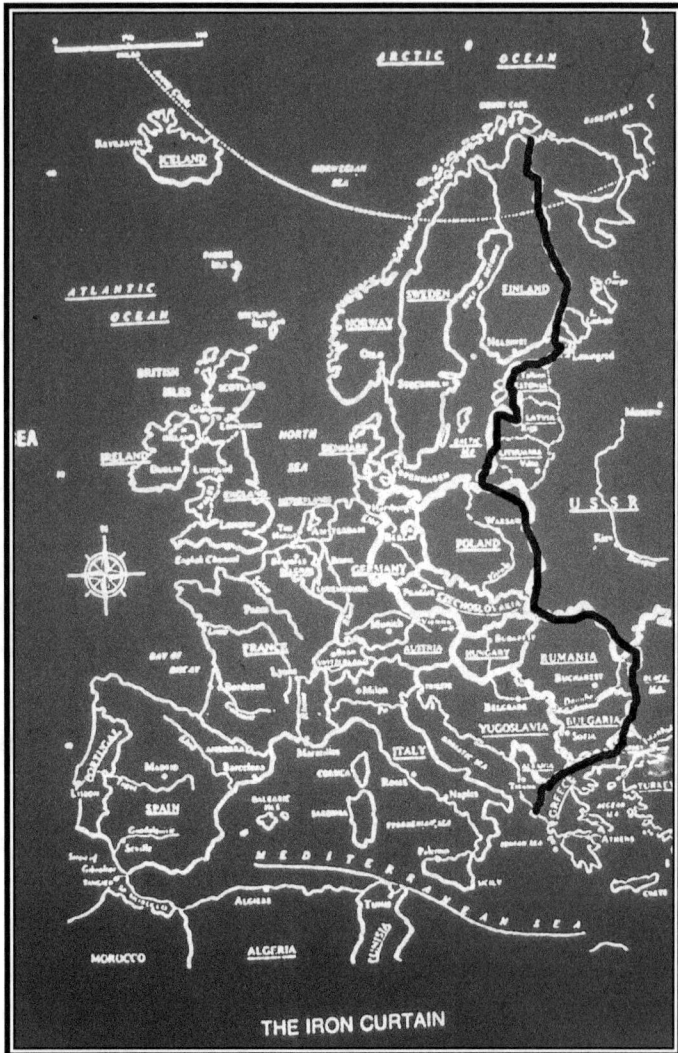

Figure 18. This map of Europe shows the extension and length of the Iron Curtain.

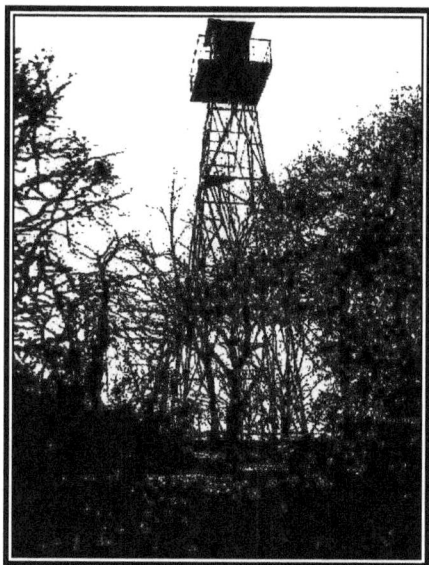

Figures 19-22. The top photograph shows a high-standing border watchtower. The two bottom left diagrams reveal the design of the seventy centimeter barbed wire fences with high posts. The blueprint of the the Iron Curtain is reproduced on the bottom right.

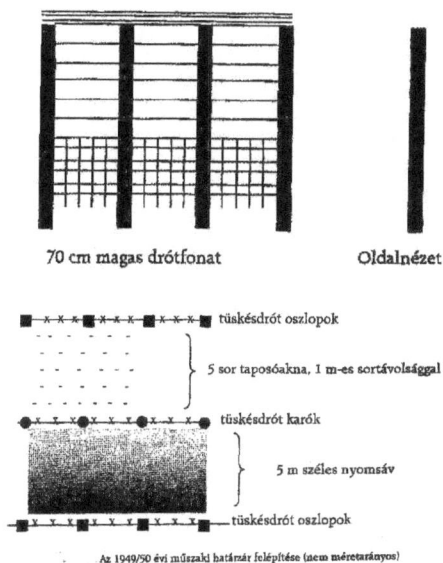

70 cm magas drótfonat   Oldalnézet

tüskésdrót oszlopok

5 sor taposóakna, 1 m-es sortávolsággal

tüskésdrót karók

5 m széles nyomsáv

tüskésdrót oszlopok

Az 1949/50 évi műszaki határzár felépítése (nem méretarányos)

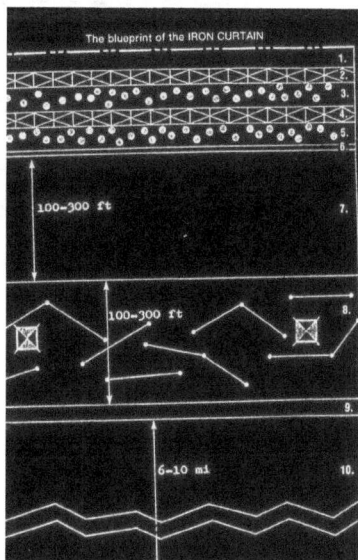

The blueprint of the IRON CURTAIN

100-300 ft

100-300 ft

6-10 mi

Hungary became the East German peoples' holiday territory. It was more progressive, economically advanced, and cheaper. It possessed excellent summer resorts and vacation spots. On June 12, 1987, President Reagan delivered his Berlin wall speech at the Brandenburg Gate in Berlin, "Mr. Gorbachev, tear down this wall!" (http://www. americanrhetoric.com/speeches/ronaldreaganbrandenburggate.htm) The Wall stood for another two years until the great number of East German vacationers in Hungary became a "problem." Thousands of them were waiting in camps in Hungary to cross the border to the West, to Austria. Moscow delivered an ultimatum to the Hungarian government and insisted on keeping the Iron Curtain untouched and closed.

On June 27, 1989, the Hungarian authorities ordered the opening of the gates of the Iron Curtain between Hungary and Austria, in spite of the Soviet ultimatum. East German people crossed from Hungary into Austria and thereby to freedom. The Berlin Wall finally fully opened and came down on November 9, 1989. Helmut Kohl, German Chancellor (1982-1998) at the time, remarked, "There was Hungarian soil under the Wall."

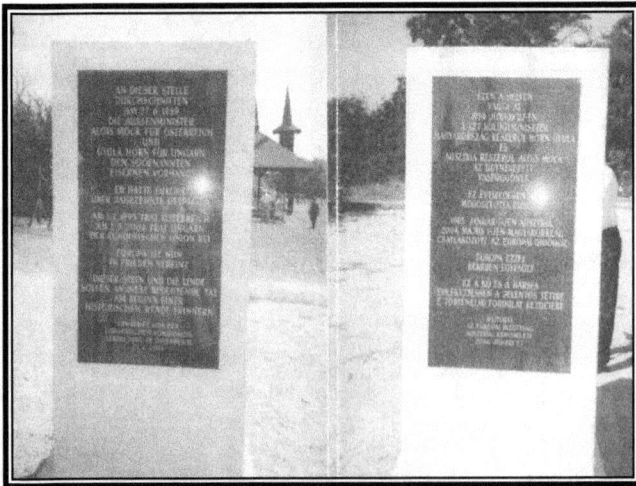

Figure 23. On June 27, 1989, the gates of the Iron Curtain between Hungary and Austria were opened. Memorials were erected at this border.

The idea or the principle of the "Iron Curtain" (i.e. living behind prison "bars") made us feel like physical, psychological, and mental prisoners, condemning us to a cruel world. It may be hard to understand it today—I am sure! The book written by Anne Applebaum, *The Iron Curtain,* is an authoritative study of Stalinization during this period of history.

Several years before the Iron Curtain fell, already on the West side of it, I decided that I would show the physical reality of the Curtain to my children. In 1982, I participated in a Dragon class sailboat regatta in Travemünde, West Germany, close to Lübeck, also in West Germany.

One of the few rivers that flows north, the Trave River enters the Baltic Sea at the point where the Iron Curtain starts on the other side of the riverbank. The division between East and West Germany was marked by yellow buoys. If one sailed inside the buoys, an East German police boat would appear, confiscate the boat, and put its sailors into jail until the East German government received a ransom to free the trespassers. During the regatta, while sailing in the mouth of the Trave River, my crew and I had to carefully watch the buoys in order to keep the buoys to our right and thus stay in West Germany. This added an additional challenge to our racing endeavors.

One evening, we took the ferry across the mouth of the Trave River and walked on the beach on the West German side to the "no man's land" of the border between West and East Germany. Signs declaring "Halt! Hier ist die Grenze!" (Stop! Here is the border!) warned us to not walk any further. Luckily, we knew some German and understood the warning on the signs! We could see the watchtowers in the distance and the yellow buoys in the water. Automatic guns would have fired if we crossed into the range of the border, and ground mines would have exploded. Border guards were on alert at all times.

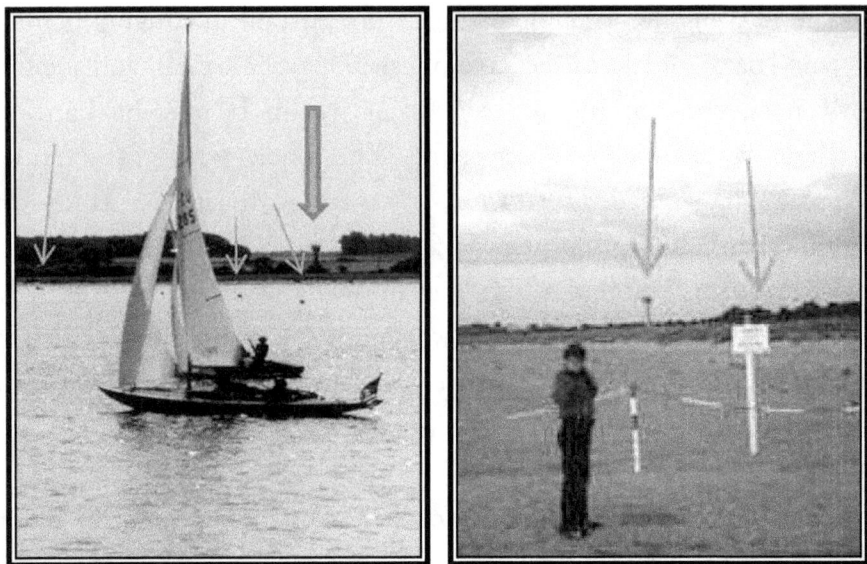

Figures 24-25. Photographs of the border between West and East Germany: Travemünde, West Germany. The border watchtower, buoys, and signs in the distance demarcated the no man's land or Iron Curtain between the two countries.

During the communist era, Hungary's isolation was almost complete. A young couple, relatives of my classmate, managed to escape to Vienna, Austria. At that time, Vienna and Berlin were divided into three sections under the rule of the three occupying powers—France, the United States, and the Soviet Union. Unfortunately, roaming the unknown, strange streets, happily enjoying their newfound freedom, they unwittingly walked into the Soviet section of the city. This misfortune happened before the Austrian State Treaty was signed in Vienna in 1955, and the Russians withdrew from Austria. This couple was apprehended by the Soviets, arrested, and transferred back to jail in Hungary.

I knew that I was going to have to escape from Hungary, unless a better opportunity presented itself to me! Patrolmen who fired indiscriminately guarded the lakes and rivers. One area in Berlin was well known.

Hundreds of escapees died here trying to cross to the West.

By 1955, I was certain my future would be made in the West and not in my beloved country! I began to formulate an escape plan in my mind. It involved:

• Total secrecy for the sake of my relatives' security and welfare;
• Complete local knowledge, including:
  • Knowledge of the plans of the armed guardsmen on duty and observation points;
  • Thoroughly studying the area, geography, and circumstances;
  • Not depending upon any assistance from agents, guides, or volunteers;

I thought about waiting for an unexpected occurrence such as a local breakdown of the Curtain, a change of the regime's policies, and/or a political coup. At that time, the aforementioned looked as if they would never occur.

Hungarians anxiously awaited the completion of the treaty in Vienna, the Austrian State Treaty, on May 15, 1955. It took over 700 sessions to reach a compromise agreement before it was signed. The Russians sharply and shrewdly manipulated the circumstances surrounding the Treaty in order to obtain time to establish the Warsaw Pact.

The military unity of the Warsaw Pact countries was established in July 1956, after the Austrian State Treaty was signed. The Pact established a mutual defense system among the eight nations: if one of the countries in the pact were attacked, the other nations would intervene militarily on behalf of the "attacked" one. Four powers signed the agreement, which stipulated, "that the Russian troops have to withdraw from the Eastern European States within 3 months after the Austrian Peace Treaty was signed." Stalin and the Soviets needed time to complete the military union of the Warsaw Pact nations and ratify it. Now the Soviets could remove their troops from Hungary and go home. The nations belonging to the pact were supposed to "protect" one another!

At this time, the AVO (Allam Vedelmi Osztaly), the Hungarian Secret Police, came into its full authority, having learned various terroristic tactics from its model, the NKVD (People's Commissariat for Internal Affairs), the Soviet state security organization; the AVO used threats and fear as its weapons. The People's Court was established to try the fascists, who were sentenced to death and executed or condemned to lifetimes of hard labor. Executions and mock trials based upon coercion and torture were not uncommon. Within the Comintern countries, Stalin purged fascists from the Party, including those members who engaged in capitalistic ventures, and the "Titoists,"who were not fully faithful to Moscow and Stalinist doctrines. Stalin revolutionized the peasants and killed many millions who resisted him, including "Kulaks" or "big landowners," who were considered enemies of the system.

After enrolling in the University of Pècs medical studies program, during two summers, my class was drafted into the army. Instructed by low-level soldiers, we studied defense and army procedures. Exposed to the blazing summer sun on the Hungarian prairies, we lived in army tents and ate horrendous, "murderous" army food. These experiences were not unlike those endured during the Chairman Mao Tsetung's "Cultural Revolution."

In the setting of the army, ignorant, brutal, primitive soldiers—who came from Hungary's lower classes—enjoyed "rough" treating Hungary's aspiring professionals and intellectuals. Army training focused on building physical fitness and endurance. For example, we were expected to march seventy to eighty kilometers in full military gear weighing seventy to eighty kilograms. Trainees suffered from rampant dysentery. We attended political seminars and studied the Russian language and military protocols. During my university years, the Russian Revolution and "dialectical materialism" also were compulsory courses, with mandatory examinations on these subjects at the ends of the school years. While I learned these subjects against my will, I realized only much later in my life that "it is very important" that "one should study and know the philosophy and doctrines of one's adversaries." These studies made me understand situations that are strange even for today's politicians. Today, our politicians are ignorant of party doctrines, "anatomies" of revolutions, and class systems in different nations. They lack knowledge of the roles played by the members of the masses, who belong to the proletariats and the aristocracies.

Today, political literacy even among educated individuals is very low in many Western countries including the United States. Mao Tsetung's "Little Red Book" should be mandatory reading. It is one document that helps us understand modern Chinese policies. The "sacred" text of Islam, the Koran, also should be taught in economic and political university courses. Had the Hungarian people been cognizant before World War II of Germany's (i.e. Hitler's) expansion policy, Hungary could have avoided again siding with a losing power during World War II, and the political fate of the country would have been very different, as my Uncle Ivan tried to argue in his *Gray Book*, published in multiple languages in 1939.

The Soviet communist dictatorship, which was doctrinal and military in its natures, lasted fifty years and damaged an entire generation of Hungarians. It was not unlike that of the Turks, which damaged three generations and lasted for 150 years.

Suleiman the Great, the ruler of the Turkish Empire, defeated Hungary in the Battle of Mohacs in 1525, during which Hungarian King Lajos II died on the battlefield. The Turks decimated Hungary and its cultures until the West awoke 150 years later. Europe united with Prince Eugene of Savoy's leadership, and defeated the Turks in the Battle of Zenta in 1697 and later at the Battle of Belgrade in 1717.

Before they were defeated after 150 years of rule, the Turks abducted young Hungarian children, brainwashed them, and trained them to become "janichars," who then fought against their Hungarian countrymen and families. Today, the training of the suicide bombers recalls this same practice! Young children are taken away from their families by terrorist-sponsored organizations that train them to become terrorists; some eventually become suicide bombers. Pakistan, Afghanistan, and other parts of the world harbor these groups.

Perhaps the West again needs to consult its history books and become smarter?

While the Soviets dominated Hungary for "only" fifty years—a relatively short time period—they damaged the outlook and mindset of an entire generation. An entire generation had to pass before "mental contamination" could be overcome. New political leaders must be grown and nurtured. A totalitarian regime does not tolerate opposition and leaders to grow up on the "other side."

What happened to the old communist politicians following the withdrawal of Soviet troops from Hungary during the 1990s? The communist political machine (i.e. communist mentality), partially returned because no other group or mature, political individual came forward to lead the country. Communist politicians again occupied important positions in the government. Participating in the newly formed democratic party, the communists tried to preserve their influence and run the government for a while. A similar situation ensued in the other satellite states, including Poland, Slovakia, and the Czech Republic. During the years of the Stalinist era, opposition leaders were unable to emerge in politics; they were not given the chance to develop as leaders or to maintain political power. Even today, Hungarian voters do not have true national leaders from which to choose. Hungarians guess which politician would be better at handling the business of the nation. Even now, the ruling party, the Fidesz, lacks outstanding political leaders.

In retrospect, the outbreak of World War I can be deemed an indirect political consequence of Turkish expansion and Muslim aspirations; the Turks partially conquered the Balkan states of Bosnia, Herzegovina, Kosovo, etc. These states came under the influences of Islamic ideologies. Franz Joseph had no choice but to annex Bosnia and Herzegovina at the end of the nineteenth century. In 1914, he sent his nephew, Franz Ferdinand, the heir to the throne, to Bosnia to appease and counteract the Muslim "expansion" and prevent the incorporation of the Muslims' vote into the Turkish Parliament.

Franz Ferdinand and his wife, Sophie, were killed in Sarajevo by a Serb terrorist, Gavrilo Princip. In an open car, they were passing through the bridge over the Miljacka River; when their car slowed at the turn, the assassin jumped onto the car step and fired two shots, killing both of them. My grandfather, Ferenc Lajos, was a close eyewitness to this tragedy. On a summer vacation trip with his students, he stood on the curb of the same turn with his students. Desiring to obtain a better vantage point, they chose their position on the curb close to where the assassinations occurred, because they knew that the car would have to slow down to make the turn.

Some sources say that Sophie did not die from the gunshot wound but was "killed" by an injection ordered from Vienna that was given to her as a part of treatment. (Dr. Janos Wende stated this in R. Parker's book, p. 173.)

In 1948, Cardinal Mindszenty, the Primate of Hungary, was arrested, tortured, and by means of a mock trial, convicted. He narrowly escaped execution. Having "spontaneously" confessed all the "sins" he supposedly committed against the State and regime, he was sentenced to lifelong imprisonment for activities against the State. Petition signatures for Mindszenty's death sentence and execution were collected nationwide, including at the University of Pècs. Fortunately, this petition was stopped.

I recall that the wife of one of my professors told her husband that if he signed the petition, his signature would mean their divorce.

This petition was a non-issue in my family. Under no circumstances would any of us have agreed in any way to harm Mindszenty! Unbendable, stiff, and outspoken, Mindszenty was a brilliant leader of the Roman Catholic population. He also was supported by a large number of Hungarians regardless of their religious affiliations.

All resisting groups were united against the dictatorial regime. In Moscow, Soviet military officer and politician Kliment Voroshilov, who supervised the establishment of the communist regime in Hungary in the postwar period, was greatly concerned about the underground resistance groups in Hungary, including those led by Mindszenty, the "kulaks" (i.e. the big landowners), and the legitimists. As the Primate of Hungary, Mindszenty was the legal leader of the country under the Constitution and the prominent leader of the only "legal" resistance. The Russian communists knew that they had to deal with Mindszenty and eliminate him. The Hungarian Ambassador to Moscow, Gyula Szekfu did not think that there was a significant resistance in Hungary.

Horthy was gone. The elections under the communist regime were fabricated and fraudulent. The general elections initially were legal—for example, those held in 1945—but deteriorated into illegal machinations and cheating. The communists allegedly won by ninety-eight percent of the vote. The new constitution, government, parliament, and president of the state were illegal. The communists planned to eliminate all opposition, including the group of "legitimist" politicians!

Hungarian Minister of Interior Affairs László Rajk, one of the communist leaders and Rakosi's rival, was executed at night without trial or due process. Incidentally, Cardinal Mindszenty was being held in the same prison, and while kept awake at night, he looked out of his cell "window," a "cubby hole," and witnessed Rajk's execution by hanging.

Several hundred "opponents of the regime" were exterminated, were incarcerated in concentration camps, or disappeared in the Gulag. The country's leading communist leader, Party Secretary Rakosi, truly proved to be "the best disciple of Stalin." He used to be so proud of this distinction.

As I previously mentioned, at this time my Uncle Ivan, who had been chosen to be a delegate to the Paris Peace Conference occurring July 29- Oct. 15, 1946, was preparing for the talks by doing research in the Hungarian Secret Letter Library. He did not return home from his office in Budapest on the evening of June 17, 1946. Ivan disappeared for fifty-two years, and we were unable to determine his fate in the hands of the Soviets.

OPPORTUNISM IN COMMUNIST HUNGARY

Opportunism: The art, policy, or practice of taking advantage of opportunities or circumstances esp. with little regard for principles or ultimate consequences *(Webster's Dictionary,* 1971)

I feel that I have to discuss this phenomenon, especially in relation to the forced circumstances endured under dictatorial systems. The Hungarian dictatorship, with its cruel means, forced more and more individuals to practice opportunism. The "rewards" oftentimes involved obtaining relief, protection, or job advancements. Only people possessing outstanding moral integrity were able to resist this trend.

Some Hungarians became outright opportunists by becoming members of the Communist Party. By means of party membership, they obtained more power and secured their relatively safe existences. Oftentimes their membership endeavors backfired. If it was necessary for the regime and its interests, these people were designated as "opportunists" or "outsiders," just like some of their compatriots in Soviet

Russia who were jailed and persecuted by different means. The Hungarian regime, even as it was established in the universities, was predominantly Jewish—examples of its members included Rakosi, Erno Gero, and Professor Jeno Ernst, all of whom were Jewish—and it manifested itself as a conglomeration of power-hungry leaders. The natures of the individuals comprising the Hungarian regime were mirrored in those of the Soviet regime. In spite of the fact that Stalin "did not like Jews," the Soviet system also included them.

My medical class of 1956 reflected the university's quota system. Some of the workers' children were tolerable, while others were downright nasty communists. With tongue in cheek, my father trained the workers' children who chose to study obstetrics and gynecology at the University of Pècs Medical School. Thankfully, they never tried to harm my father, but some did continually complain about his devotion to Catholicism, passive resistance to the regime, and his strong anticommunist attitude.

After I successfully was admitted to the university, initially I, by means of the financial assistance provided by my father, was required to pay yearly tuition to the university. Of course, under Hungarian communism, children from the "proletariat" and small peasantry did not have to pay university tuition. As I progressed with my studies and my grades improved, as an example of one of the "excellent sons" of intelligentsia—the communists were "window dressing" by means of this privilege—my father did not need to pay my yearly tuition, and I was able to obtain my medical education for free. As a whole, I believe this system was a sound method that appreciated and rewarded the good students. I wish this merit-based tuition system were in place here in the U.S., where university and graduate educations are extremely expensive. For students with good and/or the best grades, college and university tuitions should be decreased and/or eliminated.

Not surprisingly, a great number of my colleagues succumbed to their opportunistic "weaknesses" or the psychologies of opportunism. They ascended to high-ranking communist offices and some even became members of the Supreme Communist Committee. Two individuals, both of whom were extremely bright and came from middle-class families, are good examples. One of these, my classmate, did not need to end up in the high ranks of the party. The other became my sister's boss after she graduated from the university with her Ph.D. During negotiations to try to bring my sister to the U.S. as a scholarship recipient, this person cooperated. When she came to Buffalo, New York, in the late 1970s, this individual was willing to talk to me only while sitting in my car, and she only would discuss matters regarding my sister's one year of studies at Roswell Park Cancer Institute in Buffalo. Even though she was visiting in the U.S., she did not want to be seen at work with an escapee like me.

One of, my father's successor, was a classic example of a political opportunist. While he was a very industrious and hardworking team member at the Obstetrics and Gynecology Clinic Hospital, he was not the "most" talented individual and his surgical skills were inferior. He married a Russian teacher, who was appointed to the faculty at the University. He sent his son to Russia for his high school education and then later to East Germany for his university studies. At the time, East Germany was the worst, most dictatorial, and communistic state among the satellites; it was run by the most corrupt dictator, Mr. Erich Honecker.

Following my father's retirement, this successor was appointed to the Professorship of the Obstetrics and Gynecology Clinic Hospital after he opportunistically manipulated his way into the job. As professor, he pursued his self-interested agenda but eventually got fired for endorsing a particular method of artificial insemination. His party membership did not save him from losing his job in the late 1970s; the USSR was disintegrating at that time.

Political and financial opportunism also are well-known in the U.S.A. My personal philosophy has proven to be effective and unchallenged over the past fifty years. "Never talk about religion, finances, or politics with anyone outside one's closest family circles or challenge anybody on these grounds." Without a doubt, the eight years during my high school and university studies, from 1948 until 1956, were my worst. During these years, I concentrated on tennis and fencing, since my father forbade me to develop my soccer skills. We played tennis during the summer. I played bridge and tarrock with a close, limited circle of my friends, usually in secrecy at one of our parents' homes. We abstained from socializing with and participating in the activities of different organizations such as the Boy Scouts or religious groups.

During my university years, I became interested in foil fencing. This sport gave my friends and me some privacy, "refreshment," and recreation from the continuously grey, depressing daily activities, party slogans—"Rákosi elvtárs" (tovarish)—and Stalin. We trained during the week and competed on the weekends at home or in one of the cities of the Dunántúl, Transdanubia. We travelled to the Hungarian city of Sopron several times, and I started to observe and survey the geography. On the border of Austria, Sopron is built on the shores of "Fertö Tó" (Lake Neusiedler). The other shore belongs to Austria. An Iron Curtain did not exist across the lake, but this area was heavily guarded. At night, several people managed to swim across to the other shore and escape. This means of exit from Hungary and the communist block was one of my possible chances for the future.

My fencing group was pretty isolated and private. We were removed from the influence of the communists and did not discuss politics. First-class fencers visited us several times, oftentimes accompanied by a very private, wonderful expert, judge, and fencing authority, Mr. Ferenc Zold. He liked us and promoted our club. Later, from my readings, I learned he was an officer of the Hungarian Red Cross. During the later period, when Mr. Wallenberg had to hide in Budapest, he found refuge at Mr. Zold's place. I also learned later that Mr. Zold escaped during the Hungarian Revolution in 1956 and settled in Los Angeles. While living in Los Angeles, for many years he pursued his love: teaching and promoting fencing until, at ninety-nine years of age, he died in 2004.

One of our fencing companions was Balint Szollosi, the nicest guy we could have as a sports partner. He was doing hard labor, whenever he was able to find a job. His father was the Deputy Prime Minister in the fascist Szálasi (Arrow Cross Party) government and was executed following the Russian takeover. We were unaware of these political events, which were highly private and never discussed in our group. Our fencing Master was M. V., an excellent teacher and coach as well as an honest, nice gentleman. I understand he immigrated to Australia in 1956. Due to the political situation in Hungary, everybody felt weak, frightened, suspicious, and constantly fearful. Political persecution and annihilation always were imminently threatening.

A case in point: my good friend and fellow fencer, Tibor Boros was arrested after we returned home from a fencing competition. When we arrived at the train station, The Hungarian Secret Police (AVO) arrested him and detained him for five days. After the police freed him, he avoided us. He practically never talked to us, and I strongly suspect he decided not to socialize with us, because he did not want to have to inform the authorities about us. By avoiding contact with us, he did not possess any information that he would be compelled to provide to the police. His uncle was a Muscovite communist. Boros's father, the Professor of Ophthalmology at the University of Pècs Medical School, was a nice gentleman and well-liked but also was a communist.

We rarely convened with our friends and group in order to avoid the slightest suspicion of anticommunist activities. However, here and there, we managed to enjoy nature and the fellowship of friends in the isolated privacy of nature. On one such excursion, we rowed kayaks down the Danube from Győr to Mohács. My friends still recall the fun we had on this very memorable trip.

Starting on the Rába River just above Győr, we obtained the kayaks. The first time I sat in my craft, I capsized; luckily, I was close to the shore. Nearly everything in my kayak got wet, but fortunately not my camera. On the Hungarian side of the Danube, we paddled comfortably. We pitched the tents for the night on the shore. We cooked or ate in restaurants.

Along the Hungarian city of Komárom, the Czechoslovak border guard from the other side of the river fired upon us. Fortunately, no one got hurt! The town of Visegrád—situated where the Danube turns ninety degrees—and the Isle of Szentendre were memorable, as was the experience of passing through Budapest and underneath its bridges on a kayak in the middle of the slowly flowing river. These memories are unforgettable. Today it would be impossible to replicate this trip. South of Budapest, the Danube widens, the current is less strong, and the shores are covered by trees, forests, and agricultural fields.

This excursion was a great success. I enjoyed the company of Peter Cholnoky, George Gosztonyi, Lajos Banhidy, and George Illei. I still have some of the photographs I took on the trip, which I managed to preserve. During our university years, we never reminisced about our excursion, since we did not want to be accused of conspiracy against the regime. My fellow travelers only recently requested reproductions of some of my photographs from the trip.

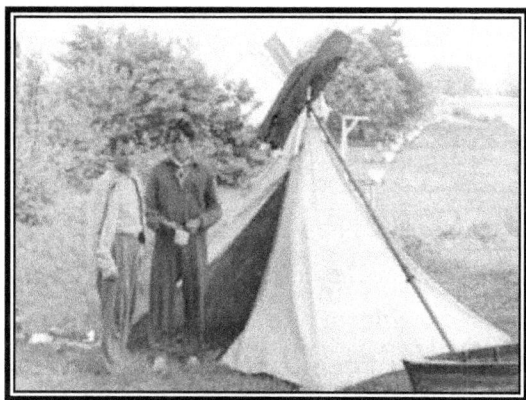

Figure 26. Two of my friends stand next to our tent on the shore of the Danube River, on the Baja side in Hungary.

In the summer of 1955 or 1956, a student delegation from Scotland visited the University of Pècs. Young Hungarian university party members escorted these students throughout their visit. They brought the Scottish delegation to Balatonfüred and offered them a sailing ride on a big sailboat. Since none of the young party members could converse with these visitors, because English was not taught in Hungarian schools, I was invited on this sailing outing in order to serve as the translator. I talked to all the Scottish students and translated the conversations when necessary. At the end of their trip, the Scottish leader gave me his address in Scotland.

Later, after I left Hungary in 1956 and went to England, I tried to contact this Scottish group of students. Uncle Feri, my Aunt Jolan's husband, was able to contact their leader. This individual asked why I left Hungary and expressed his dismay that I left. He responded, "He should have stayed in Hungary; he should not have escaped." At that point, I realized that the Scottish group for which I had served as translator when it visited the University of Pècs was comprised of communist students and teachers.

I had had enough of them!

In my "spare" time as a medical student, I regularly worked in the laboratory of the Pathophysiology Department, which was directed by one of my professors, Dr. Szilard Donhoffer. Dr. Donhoffer was a brilliant thinker, dreaded examiner—once he flunked eight of the nine examinees at one time—a good researcher, and a kind doctor. He was the doctor –risking his job and his family's safety—who cared for my great uncle, Reverend Laci Beke, a Franciscan priest, at the end of his life, when he suffered from terminal congestive heart failure with dilated cardiomyopathy while being hidden in Irgalmas Kórház, the hospital operated by the nuns.

Dr. Donhoffer had spent time in Aberdeen, Scotland, with Professor John Macleod, who moved from Toronto, Canada, to Aberdeen. During Macleod 's tenure at the University of Toronto as the Professor of Physiology, Dr. Frederick Banting and Charles Best discovered insulin while working in Macleod's Department. Macleod felt snubbed, which he did not appreciate, so he left for Aberdeen. He maintained that Professor Donhoffer was his most talented and brilliant student. While Dr. Banting supposedly was a ruthless individual, Dr. Best had been chosen to undertake the research with Dr. Banting by means of the flip of a coin. The son of the U.S. ambassador to Canada, a brittle juvenile diabetic, was the first patient who received insulin. Incidentally, it was manufactured at Connaught Laboratories in Toronto, Canada.

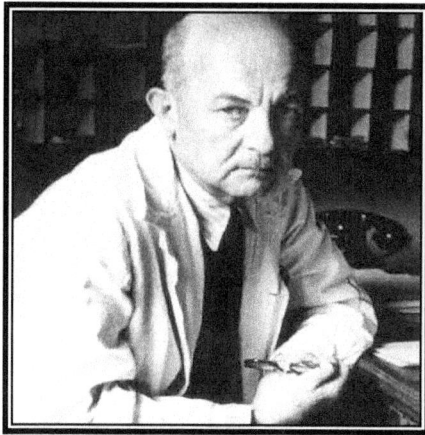

Figure 27. Professor Szilard Donhoffer, Chairman of the Pathophysiology Department at the University of Pècs Medical School, sits at his desk. In his dissertation, which unfortunately never was published, he discussed "Thermoregulation of the Brain."

UNIVERSITY OF PÈCS MEDICAL SCHOOL: M.D. DEGREE CONFERRED ON SEPTEMBER 12, 1956

⌒⧈⤳

In 1367 A.D., King Nagy Lajos established the first Hungarian university; its founding occurred in Pècs, almost simultaneously with the beginnings of the first universities in Europe, such as the University of Bologna. The early history of the university was turbulent. Finally, after World War I, the University of Bratislava merged with the "Erzsebet Tudomany Egyetem" in Pècs to become the University of Pècs. (Its full name is the Royal Elisabeth University of Sciences-Magyar Kiralyi Erzsebet Tudomany Egyetem.) The statue of the university's original namesake, the statue of Sissi or Queen Elisabeth, the wife of the King of Hungary and Kaiser of the Austro-Hungarian Empire, Franz Joseph I, now stands in the garden of the Medical School. Today the University is called Pécsi Orvostudomanyi Egyetem (POTE).

By the time I was enrolled as a medical student at the university, political necessities had changed drastically. I did not fully understand the university's complicated conglomeration or ways of operating. Only many years later, was I able to comprehend its complex nature and hidden intricacies.

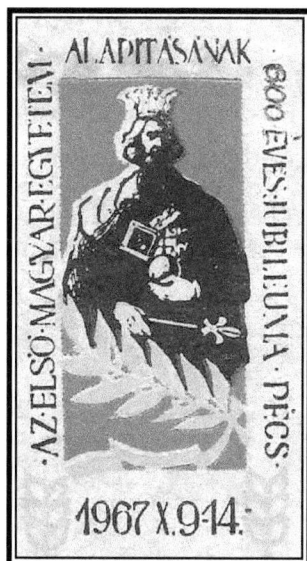

Figure 28. This stamp was issued in 1967 to commemorate the 600-year anniversary of the founding of the first Hungarian university by King Nagy Lajos. Hungary's first university was founded at Pècs in 1367.

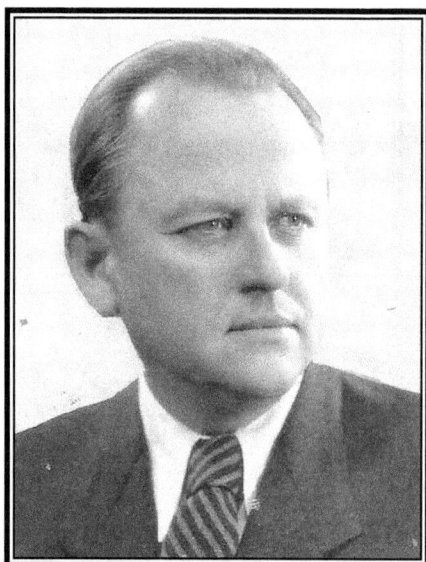

Figure 29. Dean of the University of Pècs Medical School from 1947-1950, my father is pictured here at the age of 42.

91

MY FATHER'S PLAQUE

Known to be anti-Nazi during the German era, from 1945-46 my father became the head of the university committee that reviewed Nazi activities, the "igazolo bizottsag." He then became the Dean of the Medical School for three years. Some of the university employees liked my father a lot and praised him, noting that "Dr. Lajos called everyone by his or her name and was an outstanding Dean of the Medical School."

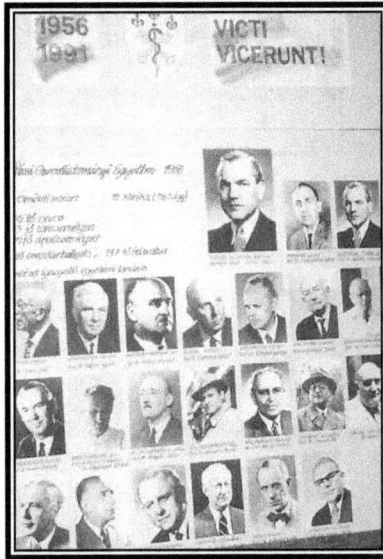

Figure 30. This composite picture features faculty members of the University of Pècs's Medical School at the time I graduated in 1956 and during later years, until 1991.

Every member of the faculty at the University of Pècs Medical School received a bronze plaque. These plaques are hanging on the columns of the Aula (Main Entrance Hall) of the new University Building. Without any explicitly stated reason or explanation, my father's plaque was missing for over forty years. In 2011, in response to my sister's encouragement, we raised our voices. We met with Professor Jozsef Bodis, the Chairperson of the Obstetrics and Gynecology Department and then the Rector of the University, and asked for his help. He was very pleasant and encouraging. This project finally came to fruition when my father's plaque was unveiled during the University Days on October 21, 2011; it was affixed to one of the columns of the Aula among the plaques of my father's faculty colleagues.

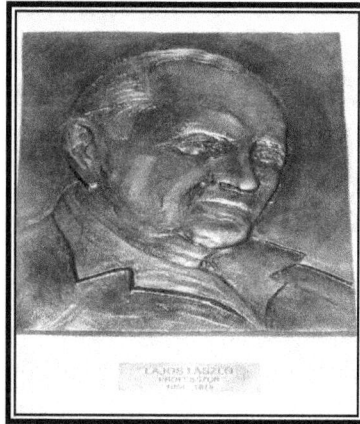

Figures 31-32. These photographs show my father's plaque (top) and the people (bottom) who participated during its unveiling ceremony in October 2011 at the University of Pècs Medical School (POTE). The plaque is affixed to one of the columns in the Aula of the University. Standing from left to right are my sister Judy, Professor Szabo, Department of Gynecology and Obstetrics, my niece Juditka, my brother's wife Agnes, and my brother Laszlo.

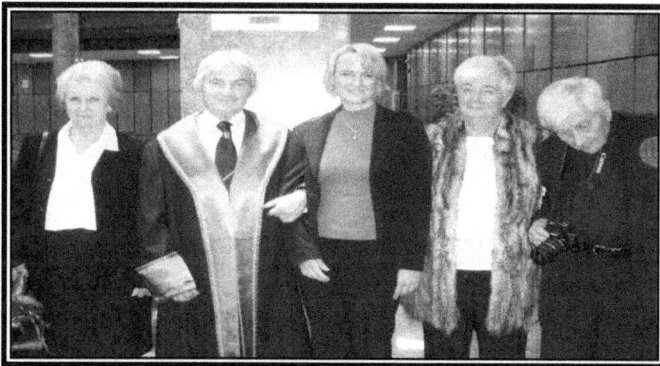

Why was my father's plaque not hung forty years ago when he retired from the university? I wondered. The answer to this question still remains unknown and a mystery to me, although I suspect that my father's staunch behavior and anticommunist attitude may explain the omission!

After World War II, most of the Nazi sympathizers left Hungary. They withdrew with the German troops, trying to escape from the Russian invaders: Professors Neuber, Zechmeister, Albrecht, Pal, and others departed. The "clearance" for these individuals to leave the country easily was obtained. Some of my teachers came back from Germany: Professors Szentágothai, Donhoffer, Romhányi, and others. These individuals who repatriated were employed and appointed to the newly emptied professorial positions at the University of Pècs (POTE). This turnover greatly benefited the medical school and its faculty. Even the political "guru," the true communist, Professor Jenő Ernst, found the situation beneficial and did not object to these appointments. Nowadays, many years later, I think Professor Ernst even may have protected the politically weak faculty members in order to maintain and concentrate high quality experts on the faculty. A biophysicist having been trained as a communist in Moscow, Ernst was an extremely smart and politically astute man. The two Professor Tigyis worked in his department.

A university professor during the communist era until 1990, József Tigyi was very active politically. He stayed active following the departure of Russian troops from Hungary in 1990. By this time he changed his "coat" of many colors; he was active "not as a communist" but as a faculty member.

Following his appointment, Jozsef Tigyi declared himself a "guardian of workers." He described his role:

"Can one sacrifice one's life for somebody or for a political principle? It is not a theoretical question! I received a gun from the Party in 1956; since then I am a guardian of workers."

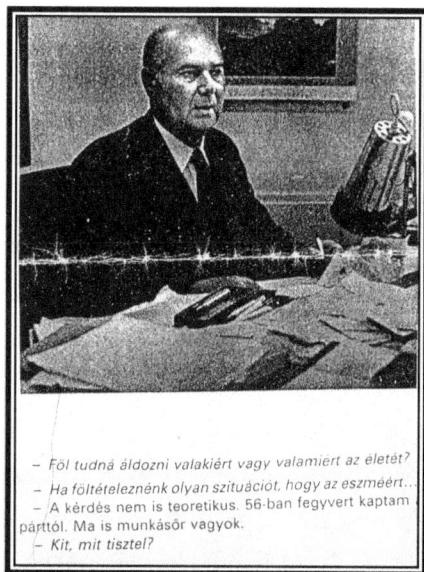

Figure 33. Professor József Tigyi is pictured sitting at his desk.

Both Tigyi brothers were "rotten" communists as this picture's legend evidences. They became opportunists intending to secure their persisting existences. On the other hand, Professor Ernst's other associate professor and colleague was a great teacher and a very smart lady.

The University of Pècs's medical faculty as it was gathered by Professor Ernst became the best in Hungary. Ernst served as its "conductor," and he wisely maintained its academic superiority. This quest for faculty excellence served as the dominating factor behind his manipulations, while party politics factored less.

Ernst was able to preserve and maintain a "political shield" that was not fully understood at that time. The chairpersons of the different specialties almost without exception had postgraduate training in the West and were appointed based upon their work and merits, not upon political "gains and weight." Professors Odon Kerpel-Fronius trained with James Gamble in Boston; Kalman Lissak, with Canon in Boston; Károly Rauss, in the New York State Department of Health; Szilard Donhoffer, with Professor Macleod in Aberdeen; József Kudász, in Italy; Lajos Schmidt, in Vienna; Gyula Méhes, in Pharmacology with Mansfeld in Switzerland, etc. Without a doubt, the University of Pècs's Medical School faculty was comprised of the most stimulating scientists, teachers, and individuals. A list of their names and accomplishments would be most impressive and lengthy! I shall reference a few in more detail here.

Because my father held social gatherings in the evenings that oftentimes were frequented by his faculty colleagues and members from the British and American Legations, I got to know many of the distinguished medical school faculty members and others. Mr. Ferenc Martyn, the now famous Hungarian artist, also was in my parents' group of acquaintances. Many years later, I was able to view some of his great masterpieces in his working studio with my wife Charlotte when we visited Pècs in 1970. Professor Kerpel also attended many of my parents' gatherings.

Professor Kerpel was a true renaissance man, who was internationally renowned for his work. Speaking multiple languages, he had many friends in the U.S.A., England, France, and other countries. I had an opportunity to visit his mentor, Professor James Gamble, in Boston at his lovely home. Professor Gamble was the first to bring attention to the symptoms of child malnutrition: electrolyte imbalance and potassium deficiency.

Professor Kerpel liked to hunt for birds and, surprisingly, Professor Ernst often joined him. Incidentally, without the "help" of Professor Ernst, Kerpel would not have been able to obtain a permit for a gun! I have wondered what these two men discussed during those hunting trips. Perhaps they talked about how to navigate the dangerous waters of communism, or perhaps they were silent on these matters.

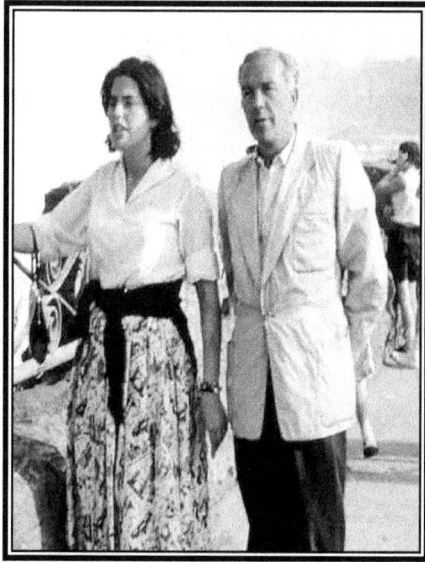

Figure 34. Professor Odon Kerpel-Fronius and his daughter Eva visited Niagara Falls, Ontario, Canada, in the early 1960s.

During the early 1960s, Professor Kerpel was invited to lecture at The Hospital for Sick Children, in Toronto, Ontario, Canada. I suspect that Dr. Sass-Kortsak, a researcher at the hospital studying Wilson's disease in children, was the one who arranged for Kerpel's invitation. I did not consider Sass-Kortsak to be a very nice man, but of course, at that time, I was only a lowly medical resident, and then residents were treated very differently!

The Hungarian authorities granted Kerpel a passport and visa to travel only to Canada. He was not given authorization to go to the U.S.A., even though his daughter Eva was studying in Boston at Radcliffe College. After many years in the United States away from home, Eva went to Toronto to see her father and then journeyed with him to see Niagara Falls, Ontario, Canada.

Professor G. Romhányi, the pathologist, was an introverted, brilliant, highly educated, private individual. I will never forget the lecture during which he gave me my first introduction to a specimen of a "total dissection of the aorta." He asked one of my classmates to demonstrate the specimen at the podium. Of course, the student was overwhelmed by this task, but he did his best, which was appreciated by the professor. However, Professor Romhányi drew our attention to the "unacceptable" mess left on the floor by formaldehyde dripping from the specimen!

Professor Konrad Beothy served as the Chairperson of Forensic Medicine. We attended his lectures one hour per week for a year. He was a lawyer and M.D. Very extravagant and demanding, he gave our only once-a-year oral exam early in the morning. I walked into his office the morning of the examination at four a.m. and left forty-five minutes later, having passed the oral examination. I will mention just one brief digression here on the subject of forensics and their specialists.

A Hungarian doctor, Dr. J. Lehotay, was the only good coroner and forensic pathologist in Buffalo, Erie County, New York, U.S.A., where I lived for many years. She had been well-trained in Hungary. She eventually died of cancer of the pancreas after an operation by Dr. J. Siegel. All the other coroners in Erie County, before and after her term, were oriental, foreign, and clueless!

Among these professors at the University of Pècs Medical School, I want to mention Professors Donhoffer and Kudász, both of whom significantly influenced my future surgical career.

While Professor Donhoffer possessed a brilliant mind, Professor Kudász demonstrated his brilliant hand. Donhoffer's analytical approach to unraveling scientific problems and reaching synthetical conclusions was remarkable. He followed an unmistakable step-by-step process when solving scientific questions and problems. Possessing a superb mind that was able to criticize surgical and research activities and papers, he used clues from the scientific evidence to reach solutions. He manifested a remarkable ability to memorize. I had the opportunity to work with Professor Donhoffer when I ran one group of experiments measuring and comparing normal and hypophysectomized rats' metabolisms exposed to different surrounding temperatures.

Possessing outstanding surgical skills, Professor Kudász performed the cleanest surgeries, and his dissections were the neatest I have ever seen. I will never forget the stimulating discussions I had with him at his house, in the early summer mornings, just before we played tennis together. He often showed me articles from Western—usually American—medical journals, saying, "You see, this is what we have to do, and we should be able to achieve it in Hungary." Heart surgery was in the earliest stages of its "birth" during the 1950s. Professor Kudász did the first adult coarctation of the aorta in Hungary under deep general hypothermia with an autologous piece of aorta.

In the late 1970s, a Hungarian doctors' wife, upon whom many years earlier, Professor Kudász had performed an adult coarctation of the aorta under general hypothermia, approached me and asked my opinion about her recent consultation in Chicago. "The doctors told me I have a fully calcified descending aorta; we must consider what to do. There was no gradient across!" I confidently told to her to relax and do nothing: "Primum non nocere!" (First do no harm!) It was a homograft which calcified. It worked well for decades as a rigid tube without a gradient!

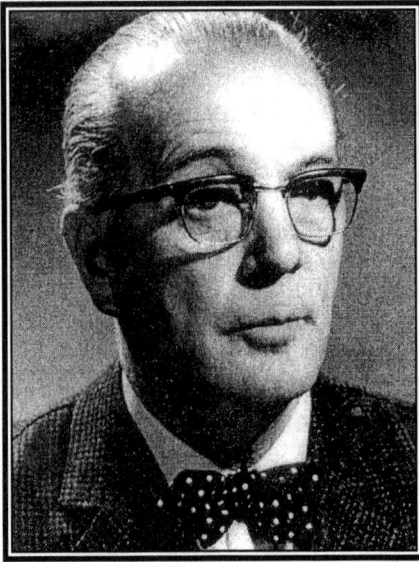

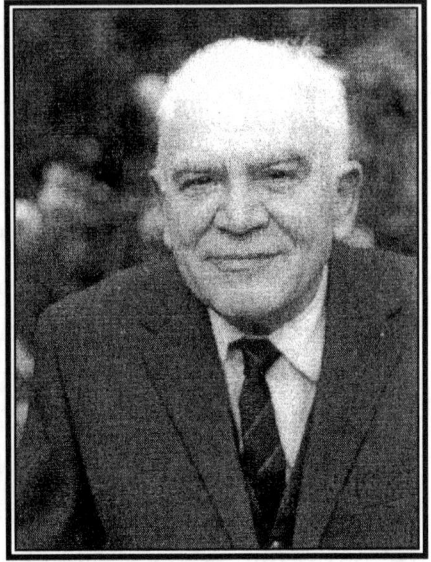

Figures 35-36. These photographs depict Professor József Kudász (left) and his mentor, Professor Huttle (right). Dr. J. Kudász was a pioneering Hungarian heart surgeon. In the words of Professor Huttle: "One does not become a surgeon, a surgeon is born. One has to learn to see, not only to look. The school of training determines the ability for the surgical technique." Huttle's school provided this opportunity to benefit from these principles.

Professor Kudász's associate, Dr. A. Eisert, did the first closed mitral commissurotomy in a hospital that was not university affiliated, Nyiregyhaza. Kudász and Eisert worked together in the Second Surgical Clinic in Pècs. Hypothermic cardiac arrests on dogs had not worked well at that time. After re-establishing blood flow, the dogs hearts always went into irreversible ventricular fibrillation. I still have been unable to determine what they were doing wrong. This technique was a real challenge, but it was the method Dr. J. Lewis from the University of Chicago used in 1956 on a patient to openly close a hole in the heart, an Atrial Septal Defect secundum (ASD). Drs. Bigelow and W. F. Greenwood worked out the experimental foundation for this procedure. Cooling the body temperature to thirty degrees Celsius enables the surgeon to stop the dog's general circulation for up to ten minutes. The Toronto General Hospital did not let Dr. Bigelow perform this procedure on a patient.

Professor Kudász delivered his lectures to medical students dressed in impeccable tailored suits. Not wearing a doctor's traditional white coat, he would arrive at the lecture podium, remove his gold cigarette holder from his pocket, open it, and choose a cigarette from it. Instantly, one of his associates would jump to his feet and light the professor's cigarette for him. Kudász then would start the lecture. You can imagine how impressed Kudász's students were! This show went on for a while, but not for too long, because the communists told Kudász to stop the show. He did, but he was not too happy about having to comply. While he was exceptionally likeable, he did possess a huge ego. Once I asked him, "Why did you do the mitral commissurotomy on your own sister?" Not surprisingly, he answered, "Who could do it any better in Hungary than I?"

Moving to Budapest, Professor Kudász became the Head of Surgery and Trauma at the Koltoi Anna Korhaz III. Surgical Clinic. This hospital was located next to the main, international, Budapest Keleti railway station, the Keleti Pályaudvar, and the Republic Square, the Koztársaság ter, where the Hungarian Secret Police's (AVO) headquarters was located.

Medical students at the university were required to attend five years of lectures and pass examinations at the end of each specialty. As senior students, they spent their sixth year as a practical year, during which they spent three-month rotations practicing three clinical specialties: Internal Medicine, Surgery, and Obstetrics and Gynecology. The fourth rotation for three months was an elective one. For my three-month elective, I worked in Professor Donhoffer's laboratory. I chose to complete the three clinical specialties, each consisting of a three-month rotation, in a hospital in Keszthely, Hungary. My associates there were very pleasant and cooperative; I got to know well Drs. Jo Kiss and Andy Kelemen and got along well with the rest, including Drs. G. Kranitz, and G. Keller, who later became the radiologist at the Gynecology and Obstetrics Hospital in Pècs where my father practiced and taught medicine. By the sixth-year of medical studies, we knew our future assignments were determined, and competition among us became non-existent. All of us intended to spend our time pleasantly.

The hospital at Keszthely was not a first-class place, but rather, a low-key institution. Two medical occurrences there I have never forgotten. The first pertained to the Chief of Internal Medicine, who treated his patients like a psychiatrist—he placed each admitted patient on sedation. Consequently, the wards were pretty quiet all day. The other lifelong memory concerned an operation performed by a surgeon, Dr. Szutrely, the Chief of Surgery. He previously trained with Professor Kudász. Dr. Szutrely attempted to fix a twelve-year old child's femoral shaft fracture with an oversized Kuntcher nail that could not be accommodated by the child's narrow femoral shaft. I understand that later on the nail had to be removed from the child's leg and that a new nail had to be introduced. Why would one try to fix a child's pretty clean femoral bone fracture with a Kuntcher nail? We watched Dr. Szutrely performing this surgery without expressing our opinions; by means of our silence, we sought to preserve peace with the chief.

By the way, Keszthely is at the southwest end of Lake Balaton. (See Figure 15, the map of Lake Balaton). The summer there is celebrated with music festivals, exhibits, and other fun activities. The old Festetics castle still stands there. Count Festetics, the head of the family, refused to open the main gate of his family's castle for Hungarian Regent Horthy when he visited. "The main gate opens in my castle only for kings," he allegedly declared.

Fifteen kilometers from Keszthely, Héviz is a resort place with warm springs forming a lake. Old people used to go there for treating their arthritis, aches, and pains. I understand that these days, a few high quality hotels have been built to accommodate people for treatments in spas in the European manner.

After the practical year, we graduated and received our medical diplomas, but not in our hands. This created undue anxiety for many of us, who after graduation, escaped from Hungary to Austria. A friend risked his own freedom to deliver our diplomas to us in Vienna, a story I will tell you a little later, in Part II.

THREE MONTHS IN BUDAPEST: SEPT. 15-DEC. 14, 1956

⌒ɞ⌒

After my graduation from medical school on September 12, 1956, I was appointed as a house officer in the Koltoi Anna Clinic in Budapest. The hospital was a busy center for trauma, chest, and heart surgeries and by that time, was under the direction of Professor J. Kudász. The trauma operating room had Professor Lorenz Böhler's book on trauma placed on a little side table. Professor Lorenz Böhler, from the University of Vienna, was the first doctor who developed trauma services. In Austria, he organized trauma services on four severity levels. Level One trauma service was for the most seriously injured patients.

Professor Lorenz Böhler's ideas on trauma were accepted and developed in the U.S.A. only in the early 1950s in Baltimore at the University of Maryland by Dr. Brantigan and others. Today, routine cardiac surgery still is not regulated the same way as trauma is. It would be beneficial to our cardiac services across the nation to incorporate Böhler's ideas about trauma into the delivery of cardiac services and procedures!

In my new position as house officer at the Koltoi Anna Clinic in Budapest, I lived with my paternal grandparents at Raday u.30.sz. and commuted to work. When I was on call, I stayed at the hospital.

Koltoi Anna Hospital was the third university hospital comprising the University of Budapest medical system. For the most part, it was a peaceful place, free from political actions and intrigues. After the Soviets "liberated" or occupied Hungary on April 4, 1945, Professor Petrovskij, who served in the Russian Army, took over the Hungarian health care system for the communists and organized the Hungarian Red Cross. He appointed two outstanding young surgeons to the postgraduate medical school's hospital: Dr. Imre Littmann, the Party's "star," and Dr. Francis Robicsek, the "brain."

Because Littmann's father-in-law was a well-known communist, Littmann enjoyed all the favors of the party's elite: travel, holidays abroad, etc. Littmann wrote a highly regarded surgical textbook, which was translated into Russian, as I learned from a recent Moscow University graduate.

Dr. Robicsek, the "brain," worked hard doing experimental (example: homologous tricuspid valve transplants in dogs) and clinical surgeries. With the assistance of Dr. Peter Forbath, he managed to catheterize the first patient in Hungary.

Dr. B. Petrovskij later became a well-known heart surgeon in Moscow. Dr. Denton Cooley and Petrovskij became "good friends." According to Dr. Cooley, "The friendship of two cardiac surgeons is directly proportional to the distance between the two of them."

Interestingly, both of Dr. Petrovskij's attending surgeons escaped to the West after the Hungarian Revolution. Dr. Robicsek became famous through the Sanger Clinic in Charlotte, North Carolina, while Dr. Littmann unsuccessfully tried to absorb Western ideas, traditions, and training practices. Failing to assimilate, after several years, Dr. Littmann returned to Hungary. Now Dr. Littmann's son, who is a cardiologist, belongs to Dr. Robicsek's practice group.

THE HUNGARIAN REVOLUTION:
OCT. 22- NOV. 4, 1956

Why did the Hungarian Revolution erupt in October 1956? I often think about the answer to this question but still do not have a sound explanation.

Revolutions have different precipitators. Oftentimes, basic demands may be the same. The goal may be to change the existing system by revolutionary means. The goal instantly may be achievable with a victorious revolution!

In the case of the Hungarian Revolution of 1956, I suspect that Hungarians primarily were rebelling against Soviet-enforced intellectual "slavery and isolation" as well as the presence of Russian troops! For years, dissatisfaction had been simmering beneath the surface of everyday affairs. Freedoms involving speaking, writing, and traveling were severely restricted by the regime. The arts and sciences were distorted to conform to the communist doctrines. The secret police (AVO) enforced the regime's priorities. People often were imprisoned and executed without trials; their families suffered retributions. Traveling to the West was curtailed while limited travel was permitted behind the Iron Curtain. As I mentioned previously, the only way my mother and I could travel to Prague for a two-day vacation was to accompany the Hungarian soccer team, as supporters. We toured Prague for two days but never went to see the soccer game, because supporting it was merely our pretext for traveling.

While the impetus for the Hungarian Revolution may remain partially undetermined, the timing of a revolution also was a big issue. The main objectives to force the Soviets from Hungary and change the system had existed for years since the Soviets "liberated" Hungary in 1946. "Russians go home!" was a longstanding, very popular slogan and sentiment. The Hungarian Revolution may have occurred because the Soviet dictatorship eased somewhat after Stalin's death and lessened its control over the satellite nations. The revolutionaries may have perceived Stalin's death as an opportunity to overthrow the communist regime in Hungary.

When Stalin died in 1953, the Soviet leadership was in turmoil until Nikita Khrushchev assumed power. In 1956, a period of "melting" occurred in Hungarian social and political affairs. The Hungarian government may have been perceived as more sympathetic and responsive than the previous governments had been.

On the brisk autumn afternoon of October 23, 1956, crowds gathered in the National Museum Square, the Parliament Square, and the Heroes Square (Hősok tere) for peaceful demonstrations. They started to recite the famous Hungarian poet Sándor Petőfi's "Talpra Magyar, hi a haza, itt az ido most vagy soha!" "Rise Hungarians, the country is calling you, the time has arrived, now or never."

As poet Petőfi recited his poem at the beginning of the Hungarian Revolution of 1848 against the Habsburgs, revolutionaries in 1956 similarly did, recreating a familiar scenario. This time, university students and opposition groups organized the mass demonstrations. The demonstrators knew what they wanted from the government and for the country.

Not on call that fateful day, on the way home from the hospital to my grandparents' flat at Raday u. 30., I passed by the Museum Square and briefly joined the protesters, who walked into the night over ten to fifteen kilometers through Pest. The demonstrators peacefully gained control of the main radio station, and they set forth their demands in a Manifesto (see Appendix 3). Political leaders responded in confused and disorganized ways.

The recently appointed Prime Minister of Hungary, I. Nagy, a communist leader, had just returned from a wine tasting trip in the countryside; upon his arrival in Budapest, he delivered a weak and confused speech to the demonstrators. The Hungarian secret police (AVO) placed its men in the streets to establish law and order. Being notoriously "trigger happy," the policemen started to fire into the crowd at the Parliament Square, causing innumerable injuries and deaths. Their actions incited the demonstrators to further resist and escalate their resistance efforts. Violent confrontations ensued. From this point onward, a return to peaceful demonstrations was unfathomable and highly unlikely.

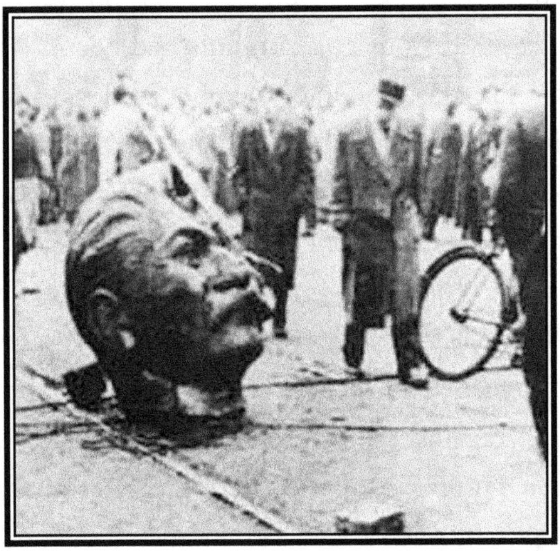

Figure 37. During the uprisings of October 1956, the demonstrators decapitated and ridiculed Stalin's statue.

The next day, on October 24, the demonstrators pulled down Stalin's huge statue by attaching wires to its head followed by sawing through its legs. A major historical event unfolded: violence was answered with violence. The mob started to attack the remaining Soviet tanks, and the fight began.

The regime was shaken, at least for a few days—twelve days to be exact. During this time, the Hungarian army refused to shoot at the crowd. Divided by its call of duty to the regime and its allegiances to the Hungarian people, the army began to disintegrate as many of its members defected to the side of the demonstrators. General Maleter became the demonstrators' military hero; he headed the demonstrators' army and took by force the barracks at Üllői Ot. Demonstrators attacked the Soviet tanks with "Molotov cocktails." I should mention that this term was coined during this time in Hungary. Consequently, Soviet tanks burned and were removed from action, not only in Budapest but also in the bigger cities of Hungary. The Austro-Hungarian part of the Iron Curtain was dismantled, thereby opening the border for the first time in eight years and enabling unobstructed passage from Eastern Europe to the West. Political prisoners were freed, including Cardinal Mindszenty. A temporary government was established while the Soviets appeared to temporarily withdraw from Hungary.

On October 24, I went to the hospital, where I got "stuck." Because more and more injured people were being admitted to the hospital, we operated around the clock, day into night and night into day. Working in almost complete isolation, we knew little about what was occurring in the city and country and gained bits of information only from the news or the people who managed to go home from the hospital.

The fiercest battle raged next to us, on Köztársaság (Republic) Square, where the revolutionaries attacked the last stronghold of the State Security Department, the AVO (Allam Vedelmi Osztaly) headquarters on the other side of the square. The AVO was based and organized on the pattern of the KGB, the Soviet Union's secret police. The revolutionaries fought with guns, grenades, Molotov cocktails, and cannons, while the AVO used cannons and machine guns. This battle lasted over twenty-four hours. At its end, the multi-story AVO headquarters was destroyed. The revolutionaries seized the weapons from inside the building and executed their opponents by hanging them from trees. Both sides suffered severe, bloody casualties. At intervals, during breaks when we were not operating on injured persons, doctors and medical staff watched the horrific battle from the upstairs windows of the hospital.

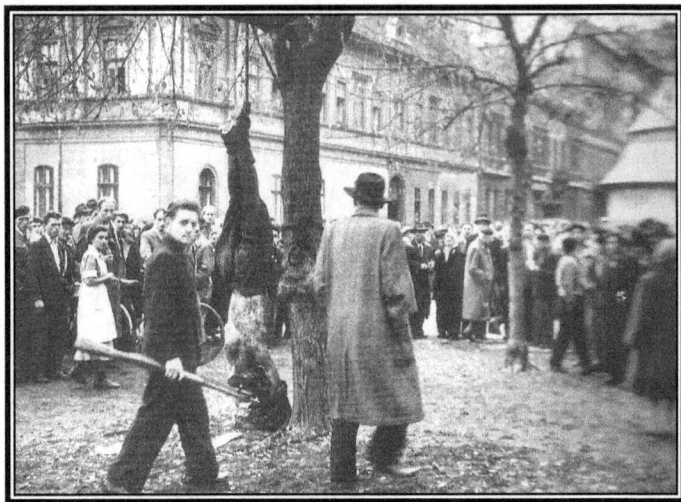

Figure 38. The headquarters of the Secret Police (AVO) was taken by the revolutionaries. The captured individuals were hung upside down.

At night the ambulance returned to the hospital bringing in several badly injured secret policemen for medical care. One of them had been shot multiple times in his abdomen and leg, which barely hung by the skin. During surgery, we found that this individual's gut was perforated by seven gunshot holes. Why an uneven number? That was a mystery! He managed to survive, and a few months later his story was featured in the communist newspapers. Standing on one leg, he vowed to seek "revenge" against all revolutionary individuals.

After a few, very intense work days, I was given some time off and returned home to Raday utca. Thank God, my grandparents and great aunt (Erzsike Néni) were all right. My father came to visit us, having caught a ride to Budapest by means of a truck from Pècs, where similar uprisings and events had erupted. Like those in Budapest, the revolutionaries in Pècs temporarily uprooted the AVO and Soviets from the city.

After the initial uprisings in October 1956, the political environment of the country remained somewhat volatile but seemed to have stabilized. Hundreds of youth retreated to the Mecsek Mountains north of the city of Pècs to resist the Soviets. The Soviets gradually apprehended these people and killed them or deported them to the Gulag without legal proceedings or trials. The atmosphere cleared somewhat, and the anxiety felt by many Hungarians began to diminish.

On my way to the hospital one day, I met my great friend Dr. Kálmán Majorossy. Talking for awhile, we exchanged some stories pertaining to our experiences during the uprisings. I remember we both agreed that if the country remained free from the communists and Soviets and their influences, there would not be any reason to leave the country and/or escape to the West. The Iron Curtain remained open for a while.

Forty years later, Mr. Gorbachev aptly observed, "It is easy to start a revolution, but almost impossible to stop it!" How true! In 1848, Franz Joseph I suppressed the Kossuth Revolution with the assistance of the Russian troops he requested. After the successful onset of the Hungarian Revolution in October 1956, the Soviet regime would have to use brutal means to stop the revolution. Tanks, weapons, armies, and tyrannical methods would serve as its weapons only twelve days after the revolution began.

RETRIBUTION OF THE SOVIETS: SOVIET TANKS, NOVEMBER 4, 1956

᠆᠊᠊᠍᠍᠍᠍᠍᠍᠍᠍᠍᠍᠍

On Sunday morning November 4, 1956, around 6 a.m., I awoke to the sound of gunshots, cannons being fired, and other explosions. What was going on? At the hospital, where I was working, I discovered a hole through the window of the duty room on the third floor, with radial tears on the glass. When I removed myself from the bed in which I was sleeping, I noted a hole on the wall right above where my head had rested on the pillow. My guardian angel had saved me!

Shortly thereafter, it became obvious that the Soviets were attacking Hungary. The Warsaw Pact nations and the Soviets organized and shipped troops and tanks with full attack gear to Hungary to defeat the revolution. Khrushchev quickly had visited aligned nations before the Soviets attacked. He had mobilized the Warsaw Pact nations to turn against Hungary. He acted very fast, sending Yuri Andropov and Michael Suslov immediately to Hungary to stabilize the communist regime. This pattern of leadership was very typical: one official was in charge

(Andropov) while the other one (Suslov) accompanied his comrade as the deputy of the Party, responsible for its ideology. Andropov and Suslov succeeded in Hungary within a week.

When the Soviets moved troops and tanks into Hungary, the soldiers comprising their armed forces had no idea where they were and against whom they were fighting: some of these men were from Mongolia and others were from the far distant regions of USSR. The Soviet retaliation was violent and bloody.

From the hospital's windows, we could see long lines of heavily guarded people being led to the Keleti Pályaudvar, Budapest's East Railroad Station, where they were loaded onto trains and sent to Soviet concentration camps in the Gulag. The young revolutionaries, who had withdrawn to the Mecsek Mountains north of Pècs, suffered the same fate or worse: the Soviets shot and executed some of them on the spot. The Soviets executed General Maleter and other revolutionary army leaders after convicting them by means of impromptu mock trials.

At the last minute, Cardinal Mindszenty escaped to the U.S. Embassy in Budapest, where he lived in one room for fifteen years. Years later, the regime refused his request to be able to attend his mother's funeral. Finally, Mr. Nixon negotiated a "Modus Vivendi" or agreement with the regime to have him driven to Vienna. By that time, Mindszenty was suffering from recurrent hyperthyroidism and tuberculosis; he endangered the health of the staff members at the American Embassy.

While the events of the Hungarian Revolution of 1956 unfolded, the international political community became entirely distracted by the Suez Canal crisis which was ensuing; unfortunately, its attention was diverted from Hungary towards the Middle East.

The Egyptian dictator, Gamel Nasser, ascended to power, demoted King Farouk I, and sent him into asylum by means of his ship, which sailed from his palace's dock at Alexandria. Nasser never honored his previous international negotiations; instead, he nationalized the Suez Canal.

During the Suez Canal negotiations, the English Prime Minister Sir Anthony Eden represented the hard liners with the French but did not have enough backing from his country, the U.S.A.—the Eisenhower administration—and other international sources. Eventually Eden had to resign. By that time, he was sick. In the UK, Dr. Rodney Maingot had "botched up" Eden's gallbladder surgery. Eden sought follow-up care at the Lahey Clinic in Burlington, Massachusetts, where Dr. Cattell inserted a common bile duct stent into Eden. Canadian Prime Minister Lester Pearson was asked to negotiate peace. For his work, he later received the Nobel Peace Prize from the Norwegian Parliament.

The aforementioned situation involving Eden proved to be another outstanding example of how politicians' physical health or medical conditions influenced international affairs and political decisions. Previously, I mentioned that F. D. R. had been fighting metastatic melanoma when he negotiated the Yalta agreement in 1945 with Stalin.

Unfortunately, the Suez "crisis" completely upstaged the Hungarian Revolution. Focusing on the seemingly more pressing priorities and interests raised by the Suez "crisis," President Eisenhower and John Foster Dulles eased into "the roll back policy." The United Nation's Security Council session on the Hungarian question was postponed due to the more important international event—the Suez Canal crisis. Later the General Assembly's vote had no power; the Soviets would have vetoed the Security Council's vote. All these events, as I have described them, more or less gave Khrushchev the "green light" to go ahead with his plans to crack down on the Hungarian revolutionaries.

A VIGNETTE ON CURRENT U.S. FOREIGN POLICY: SIMILARITIES BETWEEN PAST AND PRESENT U.S. FOREIGN POLICIES

⌘

I want to briefly examine a few "current" events, because I believe they may offer insights about the Hungarian Revolution and how the Western countries participated or did not, but rather watched from the sidelines of history as it was unfolding.

A close examination of the United States' foreign policy endeavors undertaken by the Obama administration seems to reveal that the U.S. foreign policy initiatives have never been consistently strong and that they are frequently plagued by indecision and the poor decisions made by the administration. Many examples from current affairs point to the United States' weaknesses in foreign policy arenas.

For example, after H. Mubarak stepped down as President of Egypt in February 2011, the United States gave Egypt 1.5 billion dollars in financial aid, yet these monies have been thrown into a lost cause because the Muslim Brotherhood is in the process of usurping the more democratic factions in Egypt and ascending. Similarly, the United States has not handled effectively the Libyan or Syrian crises. It has depended too much upon the United Nations, which seems unable to efficiently handle major world crises.

Libya, with its defacto ruler Muammar Gaddafi, produced foreign policy fiascos for the Obama administration and Secretary of State Hillary Clinton. While the U.S. played a significant role in freeing this country from the tyranny of Gaddafi, five months of NATO bombings killed more civilians than may have died had the uprising been settled by the Libyans without outside foreign intervention. The U.S. administration further failed to ensure the safety of the U.S. Ambassador to Libya and the long-term viability of US diplomatic efforts in this country. Ambassador John Christopher Stevens's death directly was related to the administration's unorganized, deficient, and "hodge-podge" security arrangements that were unable to protect our ambassador and his embassy staff from an organized Al-Qaeda attack!

By not interfering in Syria after the vetoes by the Russian Federation and China in the United Nations' Security Council, the United States has created almost the same circumstances that resulted in the defeat of the Hungarian Revolution by the Soviets! Delay in decision-making does not solve the acute situation. Mr. Obama's "roll back policy" on Syria is somewhat reminiscent of decisions made in the Eisenhower and Dulles era. While the United Nations Assembly has shown that it is powerless to influence the outcomes of international crises, the United States continues to manifest its ineptitude and inabilities in the foreign policy arena when international political crises occur. I am convinced that had the West intervened in Hungary in 1956, the bloodshed and casualties would have been horrendous and worse than those resulting from its non-interference!

In Syria the delayed support gave rise to Al-Qaeda factions that effectively infiltrated the rebel group.

The Soviet retribution for the Hungarian Revolution was brutal in all aspects of daily life; constant political terror prevailed. During this time, I was extremely lucky to be able to work with as well as learn from my great teacher, Professor Kudász.

THE NEW PUPPET:
MR. JÁNOS KÁDÁR

⟨⟨⟩⟩

After the initial confusion following the Soviet takeover, Mr. János Kádár was appointed by Moscow as the next leader of Hungary, Chairman, Council of Ministers of the People's Republic of Hungary. He had spent some time in jail and supposedly was tortured there, but he seemed to have the trust of the Kremlin. Once in power, he became the torturer rather than the tortured. He ruthlessly introduced an era of terror, executions, and punishments. Many young people who may have participated in the uprising and turmoil were sentenced to death or deported to Soviet prison camps.

In the next fifteen years, during what came to be called the "Gulash dictatorship," Kádár for no apparent reason gradually eased economic burdens and slowly moved Hungary toward a free economy. Communism as it was practiced in Hungary during this time came to be known as "Gulash communism." It gave a head start to the economic reforms instituted by the government after 1990 when the vestiges of the Cold War finally were eliminated.

If there was one incident during Kádár's dictatorship that was most revealing of the direction in which Hungary was going, it probably was the return of St. Stephen's crown to Hungary. During Kádár's dictatorship, in the 1970s, U.S. President Jimmy Carter and Soviet General Secretary Leonid Brezhnev reached "a deal." Carter returned the thousand-year-old Hungarian crown to Hungary. We all questioned Carter's naivety, but the deal seemed to be mutually beneficial. What did Carter receive from Mr. Brezhnev in exchange for his gift? The crown was kept in the Hungarian National Museum for a while before it was transferred to the Hungarian Parliament, where it is kept in a special room.

We saw this same economic revolution in China years later: the Chinese communist regime instituted gradual economic freedoms, but under strict political controls. A big question raised by the current state of the world remains: "Will democratic societies be able to preserve their democratic political systems while maintaining capitalistic principles of economy?" With overpopulation of the world becoming imminent and over 200-300 million people in some countries, democratic rules have to be tightened; otherwise systems become fragmented and dissolve into ungovernable chaos. President John F. Kennedy was so right, and we have to start sometime: "Ask not what your country can do for you; ask what you can do for your country." People have to sacrifice somewhat their free-thinking ways and democratic principles to live in a free country. It is better for them to do their best voluntarily for their country than to be pressured into making sacrifices. Surprisingly, today so few people living in democratic countries have realized that freedom really is *not* entirely free, because it comes with sacrifices. Democracies and democratization seem to come with costs. We might ask ourselves in the case of Hungary, what were the costs of the post-Soviet communist regime and its "gulash communisim?"

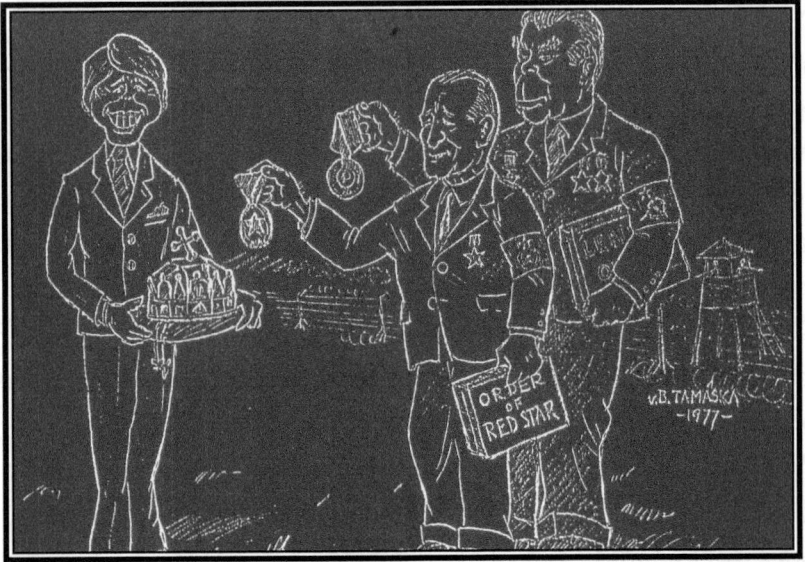

Figure 39. President Carter delivers his "gift," the thousand-year- old St. Stephen's crown, to the Soviet Chief L. Brezhnev.

PLANNING TO CROSS THE IRON CURTAIN: DEC. 14, 1956

M y time was "maturing:" my time was arriving! I knew that I was going to have to make probably the most difficult and greatest decision of my life! I simply could not continue to tolerate the political circumstances in Hungary: the communist propaganda, the dictatorship, the despicable behavior of the people praising Comrade Rákosi as "Stalin's best disciple," and those who still adulated Joseph Stalin as a saint.

My professional career living under the dictatorial communist regime in Hungary would have been curtailed. I never would have been able to reach my main professional goal—to practice heart surgery—living in the communist country. My family's political and religious attitudes, my beliefs, and my background always would have served as insurmountable obstacles to my professional success. I could have stayed in the country hoping that the regime was going to change. But would this have happened and when? From my perspective, these were totally unknown, unanswerable questions!

After the Revolution of 1956 and the Soviet retribution, the future of the Soviet-controlled, communist system in Hungary looked endless. The "Cold War" was raging between the West and the USSR with no end in sight.

When my father came to Budapest to check on his parents, I talked with him on the Rákóczi Street, where there was no chance of being heard or watched. I told him that I planned to leave the country at the first chance. Being a permanent optimist, he expressed opposition to my plans.

On another day, when I again met my friend Dr. Kálmán Majorossy on the street, I told him that I planned to leave the country. I asked him to join me. He refused; he was in love and planned to get married.

At about this time the Iron Curtain gradually was closing; it was being rebuilt. The time to cross it without much danger was becoming short. The window of opportunity slowly was getting smaller and smaller. I knew I was going to have to act on my plans or I forever would become a prisoner in my own country.

During these dictatorial times, if one left the country and one's relatives knew about one's intentions to escape, one's relatives usually were imprisoned, prosecuted, and/or deported. I knew that if I was going to leave Hungary, the details and plans of my departure had to be kept entirely secret and unknown to my relatives, even to my parents and grandparents. My family had to be kept clueless and unsuspecting. My employer, my professor, and my colleagues also had to be "left in the dark."

I planned my escape from Hungary in complete secrecy. When some of my friends from the University of Pècs asked me to leave the country with them and suggested that we follow a mutual plan and arrangements to leave, I refused. I told them that we should make independent plans and arrangements and that we should not make them known to each other.

My parents had a very good friend living in Győr, Hungary. He was a district physician whom I knew well. I trusted him and asked him for his opinion. Surprisingly, he unhesitatingly agreed to help me. Győr is a city on the shores of the Danube, on a direct highway to Vienna, not too far from the Hungarian border at Mosonmagyaróvár. This border had a thirty kilometer "no travel zone," while the communists were rebuilding the Iron Curtain. My plan was to first enter this no travel zone, traverse it, and then cross the border. I knew that I was going to have to improvise any further arrangements.

On the morning of December 14, 1956, I told my grandparents that I was going to be on call for the next five or six days in the hospital, and that I would not be home to see them for a while. My heart was breaking, because I knew that I probably was saying goodbye to them forever and that I never would see them again on this earth! The regime was so cruel! It forced people like me to sever loving family ties, if they were not destroyed before by the regime itself! For their own protection, my grandparents could not have been given any idea that I was going to escape from Hungary over the next few days, even if it meant breaking my heart!

I traveled to Győr alone by train, totally independent from a group of medical students from Pècs also on board. At Győr, I met Dr. Dezso Reh, who picked me up with his car and drove me to a farm near the border. On the way, thirty kilometers from the border, a group of AVO soldiers, who were guarding the no travel zone, stopped us. Dr. Reh answered their questions, drawing attention to his supervisory duties as a district doctor and my role as an assisting physician. I will never forget the response we received from one of the soldiers who turned to me and said, "If you are captured and brought back by our troops, I promise you, I will take care of you." I thought, if this escape is successful, I will not have to endure "him caring" for me, his pointed death sentence.

Dr. Reh left me at the farmhouse with the owner whom he knew. We ate a small supper; then the farmer and his wife encouraged me to sleep for a few hours. Around midnight, the farmer awakened me. He informed me that we needed to leave. We walked about five kilometers. At the official border stone, the farmer stopped and asked me what I had for him (as compensation or payment). I had practically nothing in my small bag except a very reliable alarm clock and a few hundred forints in cash. Very grateful for his services, I gave him all my cash. While he obviously was disappointed with my small payment, he wished me good luck anyway.

In the pitch-darkness of night, on December 14, 1956, I stepped over the border and started to walk on free soil for the first time in my life; I walked straight towards the West. This course of events was one of the most momentous of my life. I cannot emphasize this point enough!

For several hours, I walked alone, while the Hungarian Border patrolmen fired flares around me. Each time a flare exploded, I dove into the snow and mud to hide my presence. I accidentally ran into a group of twenty persons standing around a border stone similar to the one away from which I had walked several hours earlier. These persons were confused; they were debating their whereabouts and next route.

We realized that we again were on the Austro-Hungarian borderline. Among these twenty Hungarians, I recognized the group of medical students from Pècs, with whom I had traveled on the same train from Budapest to Győr and with whom I had refused to share any information about my trip when they had asked. Of course, we were glad to again meet, but we knew we had to make a fast, very significant decision. Unfortunately, none of us had a compass and none of us had thought to bring one! (Had this been the soundest pre-trip preparation for what would be the "trip" of our lives?) The weather was cold, drizzling rain, foggy, and very dark. Stars were not visible nor was the moon. Some from the group were frightened and eventually decided to walk in one direction.

I decided not to go with this group and warned them that the borderline may not be straight and could form a U-shaped indentation. With an irregular borderline that curved backward towards Hungary, they could end up returning to Hungary. We knew we were standing on Austrian soil. I advised everyone that we should not move until the morning. Some of my fellow travelers listened to me while the rest of the group kept on going.

By now comprised of about eight to ten people, we scouted the vicinity for a place to hide, rest, and wait. We found a haystack on the Austrian side that proved to be the perfect place in which to warm ourselves, stay out-of-sight, and wait until morning. After we endured a difficult four or five hours, daylight arrived, but the fog still was dense. I refused to move until I was able to obtain a definite idea where the sunrise occurred.

After sunrise, we walked due west for about ten kilometers, until we ran into an Austrian border guard, who greeted us in a friendly fashion. He took us to a shelter that had been established for escaping dissidents. The other group that had departed from us in the night to continue walking in the other direction was not at this shelter. Unfortunately, they had been captured by the Hungarian border patrol.

Without the significant assistance of Dr. Dezso Reh, I never would have been able to cross the Iron Curtain from Hungary into Austria. He saved me from the AVO guard in the border zone. He risked being discovered and jailed for his actions! I never will forget his help and kindness! He was an old friend of my family! "A friend in need is a friend indeed!"

Finally, on free soil and housed in the shelter at Eisenstadt, Austria, we lay down exhausted on the floor and pulled the heavy covers that we were given over us; we slept for hours. We had endured twenty-five years of political misery, dictatorship, and suppression of basic freedoms. The future in a democratic atmosphere remained before us. I will never forget the feelings and thoughts that went through my mind while I lay on the floor. They were probably the same or similar to those that went through my Uncle Ivan Lajos's mind after the end of World War II when he returned to a "free" Hungary from the concentration camp Mauthausen in 1945. Now I was escaping from a terror-ridden, Soviet-ruled dictatorship to a westernized free country, to the free world.

International events started to unfold. Having little choice but to deal with 200,000 Hungarian escapees—two percent of the Hungarian population—within the short period of two-and-a-half months, the Austrians were well-organized to cope with the refugees, at least for the short term.

President Eisenhower sent Vice President Nixon to Austria to greet the escapees. Psychologically, this welcome was very encouraging, but in reality, it did not materially help us survive! We were taken to Vienna and distributed to living quarters, which mainly consisted of private homes, the living quarters of priests, nuns' convents, and the facilities of various charity organizations.

When I realized that the "rules" governing success in Western societies were different, innumerable possibilities opened for me. In Western countries, one's "struggle for life" could prove to be harder, but one could achieve what one wanted with hard work. With hard work, just like in medicine, success will come sooner or later!

Sir William Osler once said, "Medicine is spelled: work, work, and work!" How pertinent this observation would be!

THOSE WHO WERE LEFT BEHIND!

⌇

My mentor, Professor Kudász, continued to practice surgery for quite a while. Eventually, he died from head and neck cancer. His lovely wife, Mrs. Kudász, died from lung cancer. Both were heavy smokers! The professor's encouragements and enthusiasm helped me through the years to try to achieve the "impossible." Often in their home in the early mornings, as I was getting ready to play tennis with my professor, Kudász and his wife, by means of their support and hospitality, helped me to plan for and imagine my far distant future as a heart surgeon.

My close friend, Dr. Kálmán Majorossy never left Hungary; as he had wanted, he married one of Professor Szentágothai's relatives but never received preferential treatment from the professor. He went to Khartoum, Sudan, to teach anatomy and cytology. After his two years there, he returned to Hungary. Not accepted into university circles in Hungary, he went back to Sudan for a year. His wife stayed in Hungary. Years later, Kálmán's wife developed breast cancer and died shortly after a radical operation.

They had two daughters. When my wife and I visited England with the Kergin Surgical Society in 1970, Charlotte and I ran into them in Hyde Park purely by serendipity. We visited with Kálmán several times when we journeyed to Hungary several years later for my medical class reunions. Kálmán finally was appointed Professor of Anatomy at Semmelweiss University in Budapest. Speaking multiple languages, he became the teacher of foreign students and Hungarian doctors who returned to Hungary when they were unable to obtain positions in medicine at foreign universities.

Kálmán's rather tragic saga originated with his family's history and status. Quite wealthy and part of Hungary's "privileged" classes, his paternal grandfather became mayor of Pècs. Kálmán's family used to own great territories of forest land and the Vasvary Villa in Pècs, which now houses the Hungarian Academy of Sciences. In its garden, my Uncle Ivan Lajos's memorial statue now stands! Not surprisingly because of its history and status, the Majorossy family had an extremely hard time following the "liberation" of Hungary by the USSR on April 4, 1945.

My parents survived the tumultuous times of the communist era in Hungary. My father's strong professional status provided some stability although not always without professional retributions. My father remained heartbroken for the rest of his life. He could not accept the disappearance of his brother and the lack of information about Ivan's well-being and whereabouts. He never accepted the fact that Ivan never would return from the Gulag. Only many years after my father died, in the late 1990s, was our family able to obtain some information about Ivan's fate.

Initially, after I left Hungary in 1956, my contacts with my parents were infrequent, but they gradually improved. By the early 1970s, my parents could visit us in Canada and U.S.A.; similarly, we could visit them in Hungary without the danger of being arrested. In a later chapter, I will discuss the family I left behind in greater detail, but for now I will mention a few things about them.

Remaining healthy, my father stood steadfast like a rock! In 1975, he got chickenpox again, this time from his grandson—he also had this disease as a child. By July 1, 1975, when he was supposed to retire after twenty-seven years as Chairman of Obstetrics and Gynecology at the University of Pècs Medical School, my father became deathly sick with Herpes Totalis and died on September 28, 1975, after suffering for three months. Now we know that if one gets chickenpox in childhood, the virus remains in one's body, and because of its relation to the herpes virus, herpes can develop in an immuno-suppressed individual. This present medical knowledge, had it been known in 1975, could have been used to save my father's life.

Even though my mother used to say, "I never want to become old," she slowly and inevitably became older. She traveled, enjoyed her daughter, sons, and her grandchildren. I saw her almost on a yearly basis with Charlotte and sometimes with our children. I last visited her in March 1994, when she asked me to obtain a walker for her, so she could try to walk again after breaking her hip. The next month, in April, she died peacefully in her sleep in her bed.

My brother's family grew up well, although his children experienced tough times in Hungary. My brother's son, Tamas finished law school but never practiced law. Just like my brother, who never practiced law after graduation, Tamas very successfully followed his dream of becoming a television producer. His wife Anita serves as the head of the Hungarian President's press corps! They have a son Adam and a daughter Luca. My brother's other son, Ivan, initially faltered somewhat, being the neglected, unlucky child. I successfully convinced him and helped him to leave Hungary and study in the U.S. Ivan graduated with his master's degree in hotel management from Niagara University, in Niagara Falls, New York, USA. From then on, he has had a successful career in hotel administration; he married, became the father of a lovely daughter, and lives with his family in St. Petersburg, Russia.

My sister Judy became a candidate in chemistry at the University of Pècs. She worked in the Blood Transfusion Center for years and then switched jobs in order to sell laboratory machines for a German company. Even now, she is full of energy and only recently retired. Her son Lacika has a managerial job in Regensburg, Germany, where he lives with his two children. Her daughter Juditka, who has a daugher, worked in various jobs, none of which has required her to use her extensive foreign language expertise; Juditka speaks three foreign languages fluently and graduated with a degree in foreign language translation.

Some of my relatives are doing well. The older ones suffer from Hungary's financial strains, including joblessness, lack of a government or private pension system, and non-existent support for the elderly. The younger ones are the ones who do well. Those who left the country may be doing even better! It seems to me that author Imre Madách was right in his book entitled *The Tragedy of Man:* "Ember kuzdj es bizva bizzal!": "Fight, man, and struggle with trusting confidence!"

PART II
SEARCH FOR ACADEMIC TRAINING IN SURGERY: FREEDOM AND DEMOCRACY: DEC. 17, 1956- JULY 1, 1960 (VIENNA-LONDON-KINGSTON-TORONTO)

VIENNA, AUSTRIA DURING THE HOLIDAY SEASON: DEC. 17, 1956- JAN. 23, 1957

The authorities quickly sorted us out in Eisenstadt. They had to take charge, since the mass of Hungarian escapees was pouring through the border. Two percent of the Hungarian population, 200,000 people, left the country between October and December 1956, while the Iron Curtain was lifted and before it again was rebuilt. The escapee dissidents were mostly educated people: doctors, engineers, scientists, lawyers, etc. Hungary was experiencing what some would term a "brain drain."

I was lucky in some respects, because I was able to receive American aid from some unknown source—I am not sure whether it was provided by the American Medical Association or by another organization. Medical doctor escapees like me received $20.00 in cash, while medical students, like the ones from Pècs who journeyed with me over the border into Austria, did not receive any financial assistance. We were transported to Vienna, as we requested, and were provided with basic sleeping accomodations and some daily food.

Somehow I received the address of a nice lady who lived in
Lerchenfelder Strasse, an elite neighborhood in downtown Vienna. I
telephoned her; she recognized the contact and invited me for tea. We
talked. I explained my situation to her and stated my desire to go to
Canada and start the "nostification"—the term used by the Hungarians
to describe the process of obtaining medical licensure and employment
as a medical doctor. This woman told me she would arrange for me to
meet with a few of her friends: a neurosurgeon and a general surgeon.
Before I left this first tea, she insisted that when she introduced me to her
doctor friends, I would have to welcome their accompanying wives by
kissing their hands! So that's what I did, when the time came! I could not
be choosy.

As the result of my endeavors, I received two addresses, perchance I
were to visit these two areas: the one address was in Sheffield, England—
I would have to obtain my British medical license to practice medicine
in England—the other one was in Antigua. Eventually, I made a trip to
Sheffield. The city is a dirty industrial town. I have yet to visit Antigua.
I wish I could have gone there for good sailing in Lord Nelson's Bay
during the Antigua race weeks. The lady who lived on Lerchenfelder
Strasse was a great help to me during my month-long stay in Vienna!

During my stay in Vienna, I found that one big problem hung over my
head and those of the other Hungarian medical doctor escapees: we were
medical doctors with M.D. degrees, but we did not have physical, written
proof of our qualifications. We did not physically possess our medical
diplomas, because the Hungarian universities had not handed them to us
while conferring our degrees. Fortunately, one of my great classmates
who was with us in Vienna, Dr. Jo Kiss, stepped forward to solve our
dilemma. Jo's parents were farmers who lived in close vicinity to or in the
neighborhood of the Iron Curtain. Jo offered to return to Hungary for
Christmas and, if possible, obtain our diplomas for us and bring them

back to Vienna. That is exactly what he did for us!

At Christmas, Jo returned to Hungary in order to pursue his mission. At the University of Pècs, on a Sunday, he asked the building caretaker to unlock the room in which our diplomas were being stored, and he grabbed about twenty diplomas still there. After Christmas, before the Iron Curtain completely closed, he walked with our diplomas from Hungary into Austria and delivered them to us, escapees in great need of them. What a courageous, courteous, and wonderful person! I could not have asked for a better Christmas gift from God. Going back into that political quagmire in Hungary and returning to the West just before the Soviets completely closed the "Iron Curtain" on December 31, 1956, after rebuilding it, Jo performed a truly heroic deed. We should be thankful to him for the rest of our lifetimes!

Another one of my medical school classmates, Andy Kelemen, also fled Hungary at this time, but he left the country by means of another route. Neither Jo nor Andy spoke any foreign languages, but within ten months, they each took and passed the Educational Council for Foreign Medical Graduates' (ECFMG) examination, which is administered in the English language. Both men obviously were very intelligent and talented.

Jo trained in invasive radiology in Montreal, Canada, and then he studied on his own for several months at the Karolinska Institute in Sweden. He returned to the Montreal General Hospital for a few years and then became the Chief of Radiology at the Vancouver General Hospital, Vancouver Island, Canada. I learned that Jo often passed the catheter through the aortic barrier back to the heart chamber whenever "it was necessary." Andy went to Edmonton, Calgary, Canada, where he built his booming medical practice; he also participated actively in the Medical Society in Edmonton.

After physically possessing my medical diploma in my hands, my next step was to arrange for my transportation to Canada, a country that I thought was culturally somewhere between Europe and the United States. The student group from Pècs decided to go to Switzerland since some of the brothers and fiancés of the female students were settled there. Members of this student group could not be convinced that Switzerland was a tough place for foreigners. After signing up for transportation, we received the dates after the middle of January 1957 when we were scheduled to leave Vienna.

In Vienna, winter proceeded to set in; the days were cold. Many of us had to change our housing a couple of times. Every day we tried to visit the city's famous sites as long as the weather was not too cold. We visited museums, art galleries, the Hofburg Palace, the Austrian National Library, the Allgemeines Krankenhaus of Vienna's old medical center, the Spanish Riding School, and cheap coffee houses, where we were given the chance to warm ourselves in heated facilities. Somehow during this time, I managed to go to the opera as well, where I stood in the standing area for the entire performance. In retrospect, I am convinced I visited all the famous places in Vienna where the costs of admission oftentimes were very little or free.

Horse-driven sleighs appeared on the streets. The traffic police stood in the middle of crossroads, while they received their Christmas gifts in wrapped packages from the families living in neighboring houses. The Ring Strasse, Mariahilfer Strasse, and the Graben were exquisite to our eyes. The Viennese seemingly were enjoying their first Christmas holiday season free from oppression, just after the Austrian Peace Treaty was signed and Soviet troops withdrew from Austria. Before retreating from Vienna, the Soviets had requested that their "liberation" monument be moved somewhere downtown. It was placed in a far corner of Schwarzenberg Platz (Square).

In Vienna, Christmas and New Year's passed relatively uneventfully and peacefully. People celebrated these holidays seriously and attended masses in the Capuziner Kirche (i.e. the church serving as the burial place for the Habsburgs), St. Stephen's Cathedral, the Maltese Church, and other famous religious places. Unlike in Hungary, where these holidays were celebrated privately and in low-key and inconspicuous ways, in Vienna, the spirit of the holidays was public and very visible. The Christmas spirit was in the air and manifested throughout the city.

My parents were heartbroken that I had fled Hungary, but they kept in indirect contact with me through the lady who lived on Lerchenfelder Strasse. It would have been dangerous for them to be in direct communication with me. Through this Viennese lady, I received telegrams from Hungary and England, where my Aunt Jolan lived with her family. My aunt instructed me through my parents to make my first stop, if possible, in England, perhaps because it was closer than Canada. Finally, I succumbed to her entreaties and rearranged my travel itinerary to go to England, leaving Vienna on January 23, 1957.

On January 21, 1957, the Hungarian medical students who had crossed the Hungarian-Austrian border with me into Austria left Vienna for Switzerland. That was the last time I heard from them or saw them, with one exception. In 1964, one of the doctors and her friends visited my wife and me, while we were living in St. Louis, Missouri, U.S.A. These visitors parked their car filled with luggage on the street overnight. By the morning, it had been completely burglarized and was totally empty. All we could do to help them was to lend them one of our credit cards. At this time, my wife and I had very little money. We were sleeping on cots in our apartment and just surviving financially.

Vienna was "gemütlich" (German for "comfortable, pleasant, friendly, genial") in spite of the shortages we experienced. The assistance, cooperation, and gentle attitude of the Viennese people were exquisite. I have never forgotten their generosity, kindness, and hospitality; I hope all those people who passed through Vienna during those hard times feel this same way about the Viennese as I feel even today.

My train for England departed from the West Train Station (Westbahnhof) in Vienna on January 23, 1957; it traveled through Belgium and delivered us to Ostend, where we crossed the English Channel by boat. At the railway stations at which we stopped, I interacted with German and French-speaking individuals and translated for my traveling companions. Today, I do not think I could serve as the translator without practicing those languages.

THOMAS Z. LAJOS

THE BRITISH ISLES: LEICESTER & LONDON, ENGLAND, UK: JAN. 1957-SEPT. 1957

LEICESTER, ENGLAND, UK

❧

O n the European side, the English Channel was smooth as a mirror. As we sailed towards Dover, United Kingdom, the wind became stronger and waves formed, increasing in size. Our ship started to roll. Most of the people on board got seasick, but I did not. We boarded the trains when we arrived on the English side and traveled to a camp in the Midlands, not too far from Leicester, where my Aunt Jolan, my godmother, and her husband, Uncle Feri (translated Frank), lived.

My aunt and uncle did not retrieve me from the camp by means of their car, because of gasoline rationing due to the Suez Canal crisis. Instead, they sent me money that I used to pay my train fare to Leicester. I traveled by train for a little more than an hour. They waited for me at the station. Our reunion, after four years when they had last visited Pècs, Hungary, was quite happy.

My aunt, uncle, and cousins Ferike (translated Frankie) and Johnny lived on Avenue Road in Leicester in a typical British row house, consisting of two or three bedrooms. Ferike and Johnny were in college. The daily routine at my aunt and uncle's house was fairly consistent: Feri departed in the morning to work at his shoe factory and came home around four or five o'clock in the afternoon, while my godmother attended to the housecleaning and shopping during the day; we ate dinner around seven p.m.

During the first week or so of my stay in England, I was totally exhausted, more mentally than physically. Slowly I realized that I was going to have to make every possible effort to secure a job. While I attended some social meetings in Leicester, my relatives did not socialize in medical circles or what I would call the "medical stream" of professionals with whom I needed to be in contact to obtain a job as a medical doctor. In response to this situation, I wrote several letters to people in London. As a result of my correspondences, I received an interview with Dr. Sandiford, the Secretary of the British Medical Association.

Spending over an hour with me, Dr. Sandiford was very kind. In the first part of my interview with him, he clarified the requirements for practicing medicine in Britain, sitting for the Fellowship of the Royal College of Surgeons' (FRCS) examination, and getting a temporary job. This was the easy part of my interview with Dr. Sandiford. Then he changed the topic: he wanted me to provide him with information pertaining to the politics of practicing medicine in Hungary; he specifically wanted to know more about Dr. Littmann, whom I learned also had escaped from Hungary. Dr. Sandiford spent an hour trying to glean as accurate information from me as I could give him. Basically, I told him that Dr. Littmann was a staunch communist and that I did not understand why he left Hungary and what he wanted in England.

My next interview occurred a few weeks later when Professor Nixon, Chairman of the Department of Obstetrics and Gynecology at the University of London, interviewed me at his office in London. He also was very nice. During our meeting, he remembered his visit to Pècs: to my father's office and to my parents' home for dinner one evening. He gave me his best advice: "I tell every new medical graduate here in England, if you have the chance, leave England." Britain just had changed and nationalized its healthcare system. It was a big mess; all citizens from Commonwealth countries could obtain free health care services in Britain. Later, I would realize that the British healthcare system was very similar to the communist health care system in Hungary at that time.

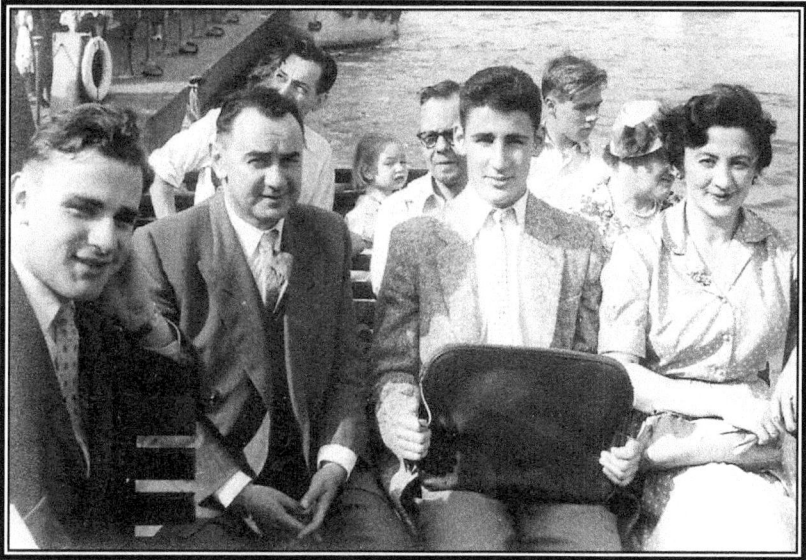

Figure 40. The Newman family is pictured from left to right: Frankie, Frank, Johnny, and Jolan. Jolan was my paternal aunt and my godmother.

WHIPPS CROSS HOSPITAL: LONDON, E. 11, ENGLAND, UK

By now, I had started to apply for house officer jobs. After an interview, I was offered a position as an Orthopedic House Officer at Whipps Cross Hospital, Leytonstone, London, E.11, starting in April 1957. Hurrah! Still without a solid career path, at least I was being offered the chance to work in one of the specialities of surgery, for which I had planned for years.

My third interview was with Dr. Kline, an ophthalmologist, in his Harley Street office. His advice was about the same as Professor Nixon's: "Leave Britain, go to Canada or the U.S.A., where you will be able to work hard, earn some money, and retire early." (By the way, Dr. Kline's advice about retiring early proved to be wrong; many years later, I was "forced" into retirement at the "old" age of 79). With him, my last interview ended, and I got ready to start training in orthopedic surgery at Whipps Cross Hospital.

In the meantime, I got to know my cousins Frankie and Johnny. Frankie was a serious student at the University of Cambridge, where he studied science. Johnny was interested more in business. Later, I lost contact with them, and I did not have any follow-up on their schooling and professional development.

Whipps Cross Hospital resembled in many ways a country hospital. At that time, it was not a teaching hospital. It was situated beside Epping Forrest. This East End of London was rebuilt and revitalized almost entirely for the 2012 Olympic Games in London. The Olympic village and The Queen Elizabeth Olympic Park were constructed.

Two consultants at the hospital, Dr. Oatley and Dr. Mason, performed orthopedic surgeries that ranged from minor to medium levels of difficulty. The hospital had a registrar in each of the specialties. The orthopedic registrar was Polish and a very competent surgeon. Anesthesiology was disastrous with Dr. Walker, who later was removed from his position, due to an administrative verdict of "medical incompetence."

The Orthopedic Surgery consultants may have had limited general intelligence and/or cultural knowledge. Dr. Oatley never heard of Dr. Ignaz Semmelweiss but knew of Dr. Joseph Lister. (I knew of both before.) Dr. Oatley did bunions simultaneously with the registrar. The registrar's bunion repair surgeries always turned out much better than Oatley's did. He either did not see the difference or he was a hypocrite. The house officers, registrars, and consultants had separate dining rooms. Eric, the medical registrar, was an immigrant from Austria, a very smart fellow. He drank his tea and coffee from a saucer after he poured it into the saucer from the teapot. Why did he do this? He said, "Because they never wash the dishes well—the cup will stay dirty, but the saucer will be clean."

The anesthesia registrar was an Irish woman doctor; she was vicious and awfully jealous when things did not go her way. My fellow house officer was an Indian doctor. When his coat button fell off once, I picked it up from the floor, and while giving it back to him, I said, "You can practice sewing it back on." He answered me, "I won't do it; the servant can fix it." Perhaps he wanted to say that I should sew it back onto his coat. One day there was a big party at which everybody imbibed a little too much—I was not on call! The next day a patient returned to our clinic complaining that her cast was placed on the wrong arm; her other arm was the broken one. "Never mind," said the Indian; "We will put a cast on the other arm too and remove the first one in a couple of days." Was this nationalized medicine in practice?

I tried to learn the basics in orthopedics but took my time off once a week to see "London town." I went to concerts—I heard Yehudi Menuhin, his sister Hephzibah Menuhin, Benjamin Britten, and others in the Royal Albert Hall—and museums: the British Museum, the Tate Museums, etc. When I returned late from London, the "tube" (the subway) did not go as far as Leytonstone; I had to walk about fifty minutes along Epping Forrest in the pitch-dark to get to Whipps Cross Hospital (now Whipps Cross University Hospital), Leytonstone E. 11.

The only edible food that was reasonably priced was available in Soho. The English restaurants in my budget range smelled of mutton from hundreds of feet away. My life was monotonous otherwise, but these free times made it worthwhile. Because my salary was small (ten guineas per week), I had to control my spending and live on a tight budget. In spite of my poor financial situation, I managed to visit various attractions in London and in the countryside: Hampton Court Palace, the Tower of London, Wimbledon, Windsor Castle,, etc.

As I gradually decided that I should immigrate to Canada, I started to work on this project. When my relatives visited London a few times, we met in the city. At that time, a smallpox epidemic was occurring in London; it was brought into the city from somewhere in the Commonwealth. The general health authorities were very disturbed and cautious. We had to be vaccinated for smallpox. I don't know how many times I received the smallpox vaccination, but I originally was vaccinated at birth.

Because the job possibilities in Canada were fair, it was not long before I received a job offer from Professor Wyllie of the Department of Public Health and Preventive Medicine at Queen's University in Kingston, Ontario, Canada. Any job offer was ok with me until I decided whether I was going to do research or practice medicine. I talked to the Secretary of the Whipps Cross Hospital, who was very understanding and let me go freely.

THE NEW WORLD: KINGSTON AND TORONTO, ONTARIO, CANADA

QUEEN'S UNIVERSITY DEPARTMENT OF PUBLIC HEALTH AND PREVENTIVE MEDICINE, KINGSTON, ONTARIO, CANADA: SEPT. 5-DEC. 1, 1957

At the first opportunity, I secured a seat as a "refugee" on board a turbo jet to Montreal, Canada, and left England on September 4, 1957. After more than sixteen hours aboard the flight to Montreal, I was happy, rested, full of energy, and ready for my future as it was going to come. Upon arrival, I checked into a cheap motel and took a walk on the streets of Montreal. Sure enough, while I was walking, I met one of my classmates from Pècs. He was planning to go westward somewhere. The next morning, after I paid my motel bill, I used my last $5 bill to buy a train ticket to Kingston, Ontario. I arrived in Kingston after traveling five hours aboard the slow train. Professor Wyllie and his associate were waiting for me at the station when I arrived.

The professor was a kind man but had no sense for research, organization, or collaboration. In addition, he also could be rude. He belonged to the Plymouth Brethren "sect," the same branch of Protestants with which I think Professor Szentágothai (through his parents) and the Budapest anatomist Professor Kiss were associated. Dr. Wyllie had distorted opinions about religions and politics. Due to the fact that he behaved strangely, he was called "Sludge Wyllie." He had a German couple working for him—I do not know whether they were technicians or doctors—who certainly had strong pro-Nazi leanings. The main subject of the department's research was lead poisoning in general: in drinking water, food, and other liquids. Lead poisoning in potable water was a current topic of concern, and it still is a problem in areas of Canada and the U.S.A.

While working in the Department of Public Health and Preventive Medicine at Queen's University, I "pulled in my tail" and did what I was told. Kingston was a sleepy town, the center of Queen's University, which rested in the shadows of the schools in Toronto, Ottawa, and Montreal. It served as the location for the Royal Military College of Canada (the "West Point" of Canada) and the high-security federal prison. My landlady, the property owner of the building in which I lived, owned a beautiful home on the shore of Kingston Bay and was the most understanding acquaintance I made there from the beginning to the end.

Shortly after I arrived in Kingston, the yearly meeting of the Canadian Physiological Society was held in Ottawa. Knowing that the University of Ottawa had many outstanding Hungarian scientists on its faculty, I requested leave time to attend this meeting in Ottawa. Ottawa was a sprawling capital with a relatively new university. On the faculty of the University of Ottawa, the Drs. Beznaks, from Budapest, were well-regarded. Professor Beznak was the Head of the Department of Physiology and his wife Dr. Beznak, was a Professor in the Department of Physiology and later the Dean of the Medical School for many years. Highly respected, Professor Beznak told me with unquestionable honesty that "if you want to be marketable in the future, you should obtain the rights to practice medicine and then decide whether you are going to do research or practice medicine." That was a sobering bit of advice. More than forty years later, I still am thankful to the Beznaks.

At the general meeting of the Canadian Physiological Society, I was introduced to Dr. James Bertram Collip, a Nobel Prize winner, who discovered insulin and the parathormone. He isolated insulin first at the Connaught Laboratories. After talking with him, I realized that he seemed "paranoid," perhaps because he may have been crippled by the politics at the University of Toronto surrounding the discovery of insulin.

Back in Kingston, I started to get information and guidance about how to obtain my medical license in Canada and if possible, simultaneously take the corresponding examinations in the U.S.A. I attempted a thorough job search. I started to look for a rotating internship that incorporated six months of Internal Medicine and six months of Surgery (Plastic, Orthopedic, and General) with one month of Emergency Medicine. The yearly salary ranged from $700 to $1,500. I determined that the good jobs were advertised with yearly salaries under $1,000. After negotiating, I accepted a job at the Toronto East General Hospital on Coxwell Ave. in Toronto, for a yearly salary of $760, which included my lodging and food. Looking back on this job many years later, I can say that this job probably was the luckiest, best, and wisest opportunity for me, given my circumstances. My luck was improving as the months passed!

TORONTO EAST GENERAL HOSPITAL, ONTARIO, CANADA: DEC. 1, 1957- JULY 1, 1960

⤚⤚⤚

On December 1, 1957, when I arrived at the Toronto East General Hospital, I was given a tour of the hospital and the house officers' quarters. I then was taken to a neighboring house, my living accommodation where I would live during my tenure. In the house officers' quarters, staff were "sleeping off" the effects from the previous night's partying.

At this point in my life, I resolved to do my best to preserve my health and live as healthy a lifestyle as I possibly could. I decided to avoid heavy drinking and never smoke; I decided to eat regularly and rest whenever I possibly could, even if only for a short time. I determined I would not get duodenal ulcers and chronic colitis. I also planned to maintain good physical fitness. Assessing the surrounding health problems and insurances, I enrolled into the existing private insurance, the PSI at that time in Canada. Since that time, I maintained my enrollment in private health insurance while living in Canada and the U.S.A. Fortunately, thank God, I never required these insurances urgently or chronically until recent years, and I managed to stay in physical shape by playing tennis, skiing, sailing, and bicycling. The fact that I paid premiums for private health insurance for decades and practically never used it raises many important questions.

For instance, since the end of the 1970s, I paid for extra insurance in case I was hospitalized. This insurance would reimburse me $500 or more for every day I spent in the hospital. Fortunately, until now, I have spent only one day in the hospital, for which I received $500.00. This additional insurance required me to pay $2,500.00 as a yearly premium; over thirty years, the amount of money I have paid for this insurance has totaled about $75,000. While the yearly premiums continued to increase, the number of hospitalization days per patient decreased with the times and technical developments, thereby benefitting the insurance companies. Nowadays, one gets discharged from the hospital on the first day following many medical procedures such as a cholecystectomy or a prostatectomy. The insurance companies never adjusted the rates downward in response to these developments; rather they got richer while poor individuals gave them more money. I am not even referencing the general, overall private health insurances, which were not consumed by the healthy patients. Is it any wonder that the U.S. health care system is in a bigger mess now than ever before?

Every citizen should have health insurance. How and by which means can we maintain control of the escalating expenses of health care, which in the U.S., is second only to the defense budget? A civilized nation may have to spend more on health care, but insurance companies have to be controlled and Medicare fraud has to be eliminated. Healthy and wealthy individuals should not be paying disproportionately to provide health insurance for the poor! Nationalized medicine is not the answer either!

While I was employed at Toronto East General Hospital, I was assigned to do a one-year rotating internship in Internal Medicine, Surgery, and Emergency Medicine. The various services were ok. My surgery rotation proved to be quite an eye opener for me while I was on the services of Drs. B. Plewis and Rapp, but was very enjoyable while I was on Dr. C. Robertson's. Dr. Robertson was captured at Dieppe during the Second World War and was incarcerated in a German prison camp during the rest of the war. Bud Williams was the chief surgical resident. In his forties, he returned to train for a year in surgery in order to be able to sit for the FRCS (Fellowship of the Royal College of Surgeon) examination. Williams's family remained in Calgary, Alberta, Canada during this year. Very intelligent, well-trained, and helpful, Williams was a great teacher. I learned a lot from him.

Dr. Jim Vozoris, a Greek immigrant, followed Bud Williams as chief surgical resident. I came to know Dr. Vozoris well. We played tennis and skied together. Jim and his brother primarily were interested in finishing their surgery training and going into private practice in general surgery. They wanted to make money. On this point, we disagreed. Since I went downtown to train and planned to pursue an academic medical career rather than one in private practice, our ways slowly diverged. Jim was a different fellow. He always said: "Greeks do not go to prison for theft or bank robbery, but they do for raping women."

There were three or four other Hungarian doctors who were in the same situation in which I found myself. However, since I was single, they kept "signing out on call" to me weekdays and on weekends too. I eventually had to "put my foot down" and assert myself with them. I could not be on call 24/7. Physically impossible, it would have killed me. Some of the Hungarian doctors were well- trained, some of them poorly; in general, they were lazy. For example, while Dr. Gartha was poorly trained and always refrained from work, his wife was a smart, excellent, industrious physician, who later became a well-known pediatrician in Toronto.

My rotation on the emergency service consisted of twenty-four hours on duty and twenty-four hours off duty. I often saw 100 patients per shift.

without having any sleep or being provided any assistance from doctors in the Emergency Medicine Department. I learned to sort out the patients well and keep the service rolling right along. In some respects, I cannot understand modern Emergency Medicine Departments with their crowds of patients. They are sufficiently staffed, better than before, with several doctors on the service and paramedical help, yet they have crowding, confusion, and delays.

There were three orthopedic surgeons at the Toronto East General Hospital: Dr. Black (Chief), Dr. Herbert Coleman, and the new staff member, Dr. Edward H. Simmons. I assisted Dr. Simmons with a menesectomy using two incisions, probably his first after his McLaughlin Traveling Fellowship. Coleman and Simmons were great surgeons; they both were conscientious and friendly. They took me out for dinner a couple of times. My relationship with Dr. Simmons developed into a lifelong, close friendship.

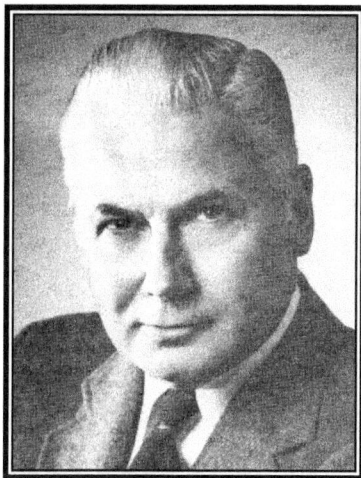

Figure 41. In this photograph, Dr. Edward H. Simmons is pictured when he was Head of the Department of Orthopedic Surgery at the Buffalo General Hospital and Professor of Orthopedic Surgery at the State University of New York at Buffalo.

Fellow residents were good colleagues and very helpful friends: Dr. Marv Tile and his family became my most helpful friends. They helped me when I was facing troubles or problems, and we developed very close, lifelong relationships. Marv's friends, Mr. Marvin Givertz, who was related to a later mayor of Toronto, and Mr. Norm Mintzer, also belonged to our group. Norm had just returned from visiting Israel, where he had spent time living in a kibbutz. When I asked him "How was it?" he replied, "Too many Jews." Marv and I studied together for my licensure exams (Canadian and U.S.) and for our fellowship examinations a few years later. Dr. Jacques Leger, known as "the Belgian lover" of women, became my good friend too. His father was an Ear, Nose, and Throat doctor in Ostend, Belgium, but Jacques wanted to emigrate to the U.S.A. or Canada. Jacques and I studied together and quizzed each other regularly before exams, which seemed to be scheduled one after the other: all the basic sciences from the beginning, including chemistry, anatomy, physiology, etc.

At this time, I realized that I had received a superb basic science education in Pècs during my university basic science years. However, my clinical knowledge and development needed further refinement. Before one of these exams, I noticed Dr. Littmann standing in the other corner of the room with a repulsive attitude. I never talked to him. In fact, I had some concerns about him because of my father and Littmann's known communist connections. Jacques and I took the exams in the U.S.A. and Canada, including the ECFMG (Educational Council for Foreign Medical Graduates) examination in 1959 at the University of Buffalo, New York. Driving from Toronto through Lewiston, New York, to the University at Buffalo, I got lost on Grand Island, New York. I did not have the faintest idea that in the future I would live on Grand Island for thirty-five years. As I look back, it is hard to believe that the number on my original ECFMG certificate was only #67.

My life slowly was improving, but I still was strapped for money, living on a $760 annual salary. I managed to buy a used car for a couple of hundred dollars, so I could get downtown easily, see friends, and drive to the other hospitals in Toronto. When my tire blew one day, I had to wait until the first of the month when I got paid before I could buy a new tire. I could not drive until I had the financial means to purchase a new tire!

At the end of my rotating internship, I was to report to Dr. Sawyer, head of the residents' training program at St. Michael's Hospital in Toronto. He falsely promised me that I would have a position there in four to six months. A week before I was supposed to start at that hospital, he informed me that all residents' positions were filled, and I did not have a job there. Sawyer's approach was not atypical; I would encounter a similar one when dealing with Dr. John Callaghan during a more substantial job search for a cardiac surgery position in Edmonton, Canada.

Dr. Ed Simmons rescued me this first time; I spent six months on his service. The other orthopedic staff members were not interested in me until I had spent three months on Ed's service.

Ed did not hand me over to the other orthopedic surgeons for their services, after the first three months. He almost managed to transform me into an orthopedic surgeon, and I almost went for it. I liked orthopedics, with the exception of backs and back problems. Ed started his pioneering work operating on ankylosing spondylitis patients. They had to undergo perioperative tracheostomies, and they all lay on Stryker Frames for weeks. He also worked on a surgical solution for the painful arthritic knee. He invented "total knee replacement" by scraping off the arthritic cartilage and replacing the joint with the coverage of a dermis graft. Actually it lasted for a while; the pain improved, but when the dermis wore off, the pain returned. No solutions were existent in those days.

When the St. Michael's job did not materialize, I ended up spending a very active year taking Internal Medicine with Drs. Charles, Cross, G. Heart, and Penny. I learned to take a good history from the patient and do a complete physical examination. Dr. Gerry Heart was a Hematologist and already practiced oncology with Endoxan at this time. He could recognize malignant cells, if they existed in the bone marrow.

During the summer of 1960, I decided to use my vacation time to drive across the continent with Jacques Leger in a convertible Triumph TR3 to Vancouver, British Columbia, Canada, to where he moved in order to specialize in pathology. We drove through the United States and saw Mount Rushmore, the Badlands, Yellowstone National Park, the Snoqualmie Pass, and Seattle before we reentered Canada. At that time, in Yellowstone the bears were everywhere, and because the car top was lowered, we had to drive away from them in order to prevent encounters with them.

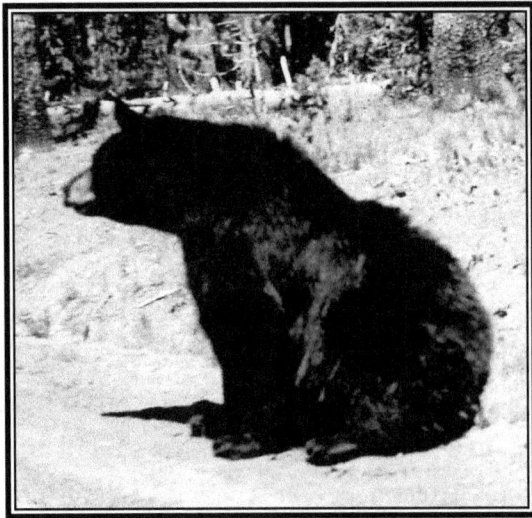

Figure 42. A bear rests on the roadside in Yellowstone National Park during the summer of 1960.

Sadly, I lost touch with Jacques. I saw Jacques only once since that summer, when Charlotte and I visited him in Washington, DC many years later.

Socially, Toronto East General Hospital was a very pleasant place. They built a brand new building for the residents, in which we were housed, had parties, and were provided with access to other amenities. However, the ignorance of my fellow residents was visible at times, when for instance, Dr. McKinnen, one of the house officers, declared that Italians had contributed little to the arts and sciences of humanity, and "we cannot thank them for any culture that we have today." His colleague, Dr. Sam Scala, did not like that statement. One night, another resident, our "giant" anesthesiologist, broke the door to Jacques's room, because he did not like it locked.

Incidentally, I somehow managed to beat Jacques in a tennis tournament, even though he was a better player. Quite a number of the nurses became our spectators during the match. They were all very understanding and supportive in spite of my broken English. On only a few occasions, some of them were critical of me; they would ask me, "What are you going to do in the future?" I knew very well what I was going to do. I would tell them that I was going to study, pass my exams, and work very hard to reach the top of my specialty, without any "monkey business in between!"

Providing me with some relief from my professional endeavors, Ed Simmons oftentimes invited me to sail on his Nova Scotia schooner; we had great times sailing together, and he introduced me to one of the most beautiful yacht clubs in the world, the Royal Canadian Yacht Club (RCYC) located on Toronto Island in Toronto Harbor. Ed invited me to the celebration for Walter Windeyer, who just returned from Europe, where he won the Dragon Gold Cup. Windeyer was the first North American sailor to win this sailing trophy. A few years later, another American won it: Bill Henry from Seattle, Washington.

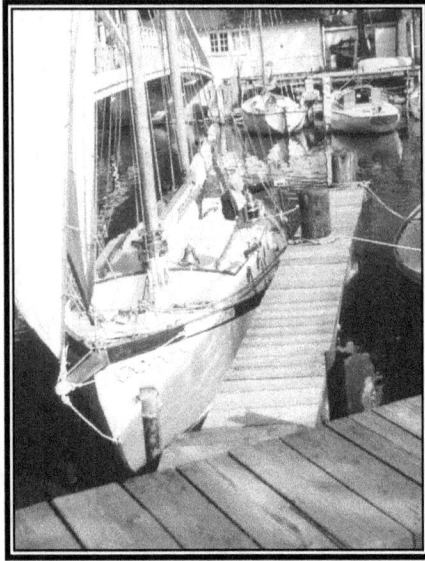

Figure. 43. Dr. Ed Simmons's Nova Scotia schooner is moored dockside while Ed stands in its cockpit.

Ed and his wife Joyce also invited me several times to be their dinner guest at their house in Toronto, where I met Drs. Bill Mustard, Salter, Lindsey, and other famous Toronto surgeons. Per Ed Simmons' invitations, I accompanied him on the university orthopedic rounds, which periodically were conducted by Professors Dewar and Harris. On one occasion, I presented the review on "100 enchondromas." Ed prepared me conscientiously: "Do not talk fast and have lots of slides." My presentation was successful. An excellent mentor and friend, Ed always went out of his way to provide me with the assistance, encouragement, help, support, and teaching I needed.

While completing my internship at the Toronto East General Hospital, I became involved in learning North American medicine as it is delivered to and received by the public. Practicing medicine in Canada was very different from my previous experiences in Hungary and in England as part of the National Health Service. By means of my internship at the Toronto East General Hospital, I headed down the professional road, but I still was not in a first-class, university-affiliated medical center with intensive teaching. At Toronto East Hospital, I came to know supportive specialists, concerned individuals, and helping hands. Some of them became my lifelong friends and supporters. Without their help, I would not have been able to attain a spot at an academic medical center and become part of an academic medical practice! For close to two-and-a-half years, I worked at the Toronto East General Hospital, where I really did not waste time; the experience enabled me to take the next big step in my medical training and career.

After I was rejected by Dr. Sawyer from the residency program at St. Michael's Hospital, I began looking into every possible opportunity for surgical training. In response to my inquiries to Massachusetts General Hospital, I was informed that I would have to write examinations to qualify for residency, since they take only eight successful candidates. I also applied to the program at Columbia University Medical Center in New York City. Upon securing an interview, I travelled to New York by train; I thought the interview at Columbia went ok. After returning to Toronto, I was offered a position in the Gallie course at the University of Toronto's Banting Institute with Dr. Raymond Heimbecker. After thorough consideration, I decided to take it, in spite of the fact that my future clinical training was not guaranteed.

OBTAINING ACADEMIC TRAINING IN SURGERY: THE BANTING INSTITUTE, UNIVERSITY OF TORONTO, ONTARIO, CANADA: JULY 1, 1960- JULY 1, 1961

∼⫘∽

After two-and-a-half years at the Toronto East General Hospital, I needed some sound progress in order to gain admittance into the academic medical establishment and receive academic training. Due to Dr. Ed Simmons's strong support and referral and references from others, I obtained a job as a research fellow with Dr. Ray Heimbecker. Dr. Ray Heimbecker's section was part of Dr. Bill Bigelow's lab at the University of Toronto's Banting Institute. My fellowship would last for a year; upon its successful completion, I would be offered the opportunity to continue in the famous Gallie course, a postgraduate, general surgical training program, beginning July 1, 1961.

At the outset, as a fellow, I had two responsibilities: one was clinical in nature and the other was research-oriented. Clinically, I was required to join

AN INCREDIBLE JOURNEY

the open-heart team, whenever its surgeons were performing open-heart surgery at Toronto General Hospital; I had to regulate the patient's temperature by perfusing the heat exchanger with cold and warm water. Dr. Bigelow's basic research dictated that we reduce the patient's metabolism by thirty percent by lowering his/her body temperature to thirty Celsius. Dr. Bigelow's basic work was used by Dr. Lewis of Chicago, who closed the first Atrial Septal Defect (ASD) Secundum openly while the patient's circulation was arrested at thirty Celsius body hypothermia. Bigelow and Greenwood had done the basic work in the area of body hypothermia. During the 1950s, the hospital would not allow Bigelow to operate on patients using hypothermic arrest. (Incidentally, I submitted my thoughts on "Uncle Bill" to the "heart group" after he passed away around 2011; See Appendix 6)

In the laboratory, under Dr. Heimbecker's overall supervision, I had two major projects:

• I had to learn how to put dogs on the pump and replace their tricuspid valves; later, I would replace their mitral valves and take them off pump, obtaining survivors for long-term follow-up. The replacement tricuspid valve was obtained from the donor dog's aortic valve, which was trimmed, sutured to a plastic ring, and implanted in the mitral position. Recently a series on replacing the mitral valve in humans was presented using almost the same technique. Dr. Heimbecker helped me at the beginning, and Dr. Gordon Murray, who was a good friend of Dr. Heimbecker, often advised us. As long as Dr. Bigelow was not around, Dr. Murray would give us very useful suggestions and tricks. Drs. Bigelow and Murray obviously were not friends due to their "vicious rivalry." Dr. Murray made the same point several times: "Try to do this operation without pump." Now, fifty years later, these techniques are used more and more often and are becoming standards for valve replacements!

161

• I had to place dogs on pump, cross clamp their aortas, place ice chips on their hearts for sixty or more minutes, remove the clamps, and measure their cardiac outputs before and after their hearts arrested, while recording intra-cardiac pressures. Calculations on a semi logarithmic paper were done and the final pictures were documented by Starling's curves. We could show that, using this technique, the dog's hearts did not sustain any damage with one-hour ice chip arrest. These findings were significant. At the end of my year in the Banting Institute, I wrote my thesis on these experiments and passed an oral examination to obtain my Bachelor of Medical Sciences (B.Sc. Med.) degree from the University of Toronto. This work was presented at the meeting of the University Surgeons and published in the Archives of Surgery in 1963. Interestingly, this technique of cardiac arrest still is routinely being used, over forty-five years later, in open-heart surgery cases.

During my times as a research fellow, I also managed to compile a paper with Dr. R. J. Baird, titled "Emboli to the Arm." Statistically, this paper withstands the "test of time" and still is valid. Later in the year, I actively helped Baird do a study that he designed: "Left Ventricular Support and Oxygen Consumption and Cardiac Metabolism with Left Atrial to Femoral Bypass." The drainage was obtained through a metal "J" shaped cannula with a retractable needle to pierce through the atrial septum to the left atrium. The blood was returned via the femoral artery. Left atrial to femoral bypass was helpful, but it did not dramatically reduce the O2 consumption of the myocardium of the left ventricle.

Dr. Bigelow's fellow was Dr. Jimmy Yao, an ambitious, hard-working Chinese immigrant with good hands and a pushy attitude. He and Dr. Trimble were working on the "hibernating hormone." Dr. Bigelow thought that the brown fat that secretes the hibernating hormone that puts animals into hibernation could be used during open-heart surgery. He hypothesized that if you isolate the hibernating hormone, the active ingredient from the "brown fat" of groundhogs, you can inject it into the patient, so his/her heart will hibernate too, tolerate low temperatures, not fibrillate, and maintain a minimal O2 demand; this procedure would allow the surgeon to operate on the patient's heart without using the pump and without causing subsequent damage to the patient's organ.

Interestingly, I just read an article on a case of human hibernoma (i.e. brown fat tumor). The article did not mention the possibility of an existing hibernating hormone.

Believe it or not, Bigelow tried this procedure on a patient; with great fanfare (he invited famous authorities to be present during the first part of the procedure), he injected the "extracted hormone" into a twenty-year-old patient with a ventricular septal defect (VSD) that needed to be closed. During the operation, the patient's heart fibrillated at twenty Celsius, and in order to save his life, Bigelow put the patient on bypass. The extracted hibernating hormone was reexamined and was found to be contaminated by an ethylene alcohol substance, probably originating from the IV and other plastic materials used for the chemical processes.

I always thought that this whole idea was pushed and faked by Dr. A. Trimble for the purpose of his future advancement. Trimble became a staff member later on and seemed to be a good surgeon until he became an alcoholic and had to be dismissed. He never was fully rehabilitated or cured.

Visitors frequently came to the laboratory at the Banting Institute, since groundbreaking research on total body hypothermia was being conducted there. The visitors behaved differently. Dr. Henry Swann acted as if he owned the entire lab. Dr. Bigelow's father, a general practitioner from Brandon, Manitoba, Canada, was delightful. Dr. Gordon Murray was the most helpful with his frequent, numerous suggestions. On the clinical side, we had international visitors, including Dr. Charles DuBost from Paris, France and Drs. Boerema and Nauta from Rotterdam, Netherlands, with whom we, the residents, lunched in the cafeteria and chatted.

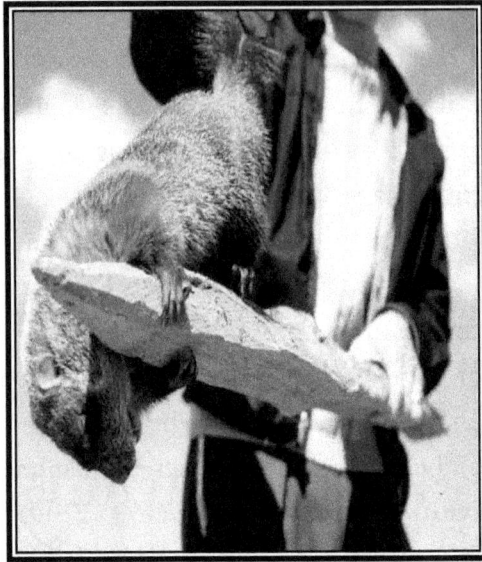

Figure 44. This photograph shows a stiffened groundhog in hibernation.

At this time, Dr. Littmann already had developed quite a reputation. When he arrived in Toronto as a "heart surgeon," he obviously was not recognized as such. He was told to complete the necessary exams, which we all had to do. Dr. Bigelow hired him to supervise the pump runs and take night calls. I was told Littmann almost never bothered to get up at night and take care of the problems. Then I heard that he returned to Hungary. Of course, as a good communist, he was offered another "good" job there and kept on practicing surgery.

We operated on two dogs per week on the pump. At that time, the routine was to obtain enough blood for the pump (the pumps were primed by pure blood clinically and experimentally) to put the dog on and obtain a living specimen postoperatively. It was Denton Cooley who first showed that haemodilution could be used to prime the pump; it is more advantageous, avoiding massive blood transfusion and its consequences, and it safely saves a lot of blood—and money.

At this time, even though my schedule was quite busy, while I was living on the east side of Toronto with the family of one of my previous colleagues from Toronto East General Hospital, I made private house calls at night. I had completed the examination requirements to practice medicine in Ontario, and I had obtained my medical license. I managed to do this type of work as a side job. This "moonlighting" experience gave me a little more financial support, while it also taught me the hard facts about this type of medical work. In those days, medical practitioners doing private house calls were very lonely and unsupported. Several times when I telephoned patients' physicians or the surgeons to whom the patients had been referred, my inquiries and findings were disregarded by the doctors on the other ends of the telephone lines. In one case, the next day, I told the physician that I suspected the patient had appendicitis; he answered, "The patient already had it removed. It was obvious." There was not any conceivable means whereby this would have been "obvious" to me after I examined the patient at 1:00 a.m. in the patient's house! This physician's response was very poor and completely inappropriate under the circumstances!

As previously mentioned, one of my clinical duties as a research fellow at The Banting Institute was to help run the pump and control the heat-exchanger during open heart surgeries. A black man—married to a white, female nurse—Denny Sanford was the pump technician, with whom I worked. He could be quite exuberant at times. Once while running the pump, Denny fell off his chair. Fully aware of the situation and not expecting any answer, Dr. Bigelow looked back at him and said, "Denny, did you fall asleep?" Denny and his family decided to try to immigrate to Australia at one point. They did not get visas for immigration. His great friend was Mr. Cookie Gilchrist, the running back for the Buffalo Bills.

Repeatedly going over to the hospital for open-heart surgeries, I got to know Chief Resident Peter Kuypers. We became great friends, and I was invited to his house. Nicki, his wife, was an English nurse. A tall (6 feet 2 inches), husky individual, Peter wore size ten surgical gloves. Later I learned he was being considered for the job in Kingston, Ontario, Canada. I do not know whether he was offered the job, but he later told me that Dr. Bigelow advised him to go home to the Netherlands. Bigelow's advice was sound. Peter weighed his options and went back to the Netherlands, where he became the chief of cardiac surgery at Nijmegen.

In his childhood or during his teenage years, Peter had severe rheumatic fever from which he developed mitral stenosis. Dr. Bromm of Leyden performed a closed mitral commissurotomy on him. While he was recuperating, Peter's wife Nicki drove him around to the various university centers, where he was organizing the healthcare approach to cardiac surgery. Shortly after recovering from this surgery in the late 1960s, Peter performed the first coronary artery bypass grafts on patients in Europe. He helped to establish open-heart surgery in Vienna and other European cities. Around this time, patients from the Netherlands still were traveling to the Texas Heart Institute in Houston to be operated on by Dr. Denton Cooley, a pioneering American heart surgeon.

Peter remained very active professionally for years and ran a tight but very well-organized unit. I frequently saw him at various meetings. He and his wife visited us in Florida when I was vacationing there with my wife, and we attended a meeting of the American Association for Thoracic Surgery (AATS) together in Tampa. The Kuypers did not have children, but they adopted two, a boy and a girl. The girl came to visit us when we were living on Grand Island (New York). Charlotte maintained that the Kuypers's daughter had "an eye on" our son, Paul. The Kuypers's son ended up applying for a police job in the Netherlands, but he was rejected, since he had a previous speeding ticket on his motorcycle.

A few years after, Peter underwent a repeat closed mitral commissurotomy, Peter needed another open-heart surgery procedure: his mitral valve needed to be replaced. He went to Oregon to obtain firsthand advice about what type of valve he should receive. After reviewing the current valve statistics with Peter, Dr. A. Starr persuaded Peter to receive the new, cloth-covered, Starr-Edwards valve. This valve became notorious for fraying cloth on its struts and embolization of the cloth. Peter underwent surgery—I do not know whether it was performed in Oregon or at home in the Netherlands—and afterwards he seemed to be relatively well for several years.

However, anticoagulation became a problem for Peter, due to his lifestyle: every time Peter and his wife Nicki visited the U.S.A., which was frequently, his diet changed for the worse; he increasingly smoked and spent many hours drinking in the bar at night. These lifestyle choices may have proved to be detrimental to his health and his anticoagulation level; they certainly would not have helped it. I saw Peter several times at his home and here in the U.S. One day we received the sad news: when Nicki called him to come downstairs for breakfast, and he did not answer, she went upstairs to find him dead. Arrhythmia, stroke from the fraying valve cloth, or hemorrhage may have been the reason(s) for his sudden death in his early fifties. I heard several years later from Stephan—the Polish attending doctor in Nijmegen, The Netherlands—that one night Nicki was brought into emergency in fulminating pulmonary edema due to severe aortic stenosis and left ventricular failure. Unfortunately, she did not recover and died.

In the middle of my research year at The Banting Institute, I received my next appointment to start as a resident on Dr. Bigelow's cardiovascular service on July 1, 1961.This was the first sign of my admittance into the general surgical Gallie course but not an assurance! I was beginning to achieve my goal of attaining academic training in surgery! The progress and future of my postgraduate education seemed to be "secured." I began to reconsider my goals and medical future. I had reached the stage when I could look into the future with hope and confidence.

THE FAMILY I LEFT BEHIND: 1956-1975

~⋙~

Returning to Hungary after 1956 was impossible for me and most of the other Hungarian refugees. During the 1960s, some of my friends traveled to Hungary, landed at the airport in Budapest, were kept there under guard, and then were loaded upon the first planes leaving for the West. Although the government granted amnesty, those who returned were never sure what they might have to endure.

In 1963, my mother visited me in Toronto for the first time since 1956. I will discuss the circumstances of her visit later in another chapter. Charlotte met my brother Laci and his wife Agnes for the first time, when we went to a ski resort at St. Anton, Austria, in 1970 with the Buffalo General Hospital group. My brother and Agnes came and stayed with us.

I never had a second thought to permanently return to Hungary, but I wanted to see my relatives in a few years, which did not happen until 1972. By that time, my grandparents on both sides of the family had died. Professor Antoine at the University of Vienna invited my father to give a visiting lecture. My father's lecture was not the best—he gave it using a mixture of German and English—but my parents were treated royally. This opportunity afforded my family the chance to visit with my parents.

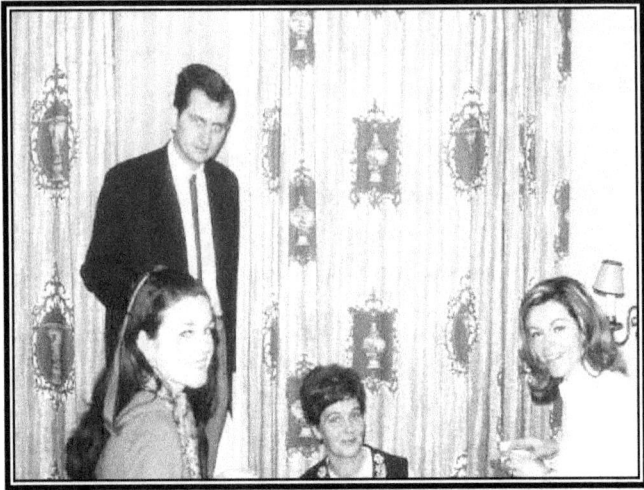

Figure 45. My brother Lacko (standing), Charlotte's sister Cathy (left), Lacko's wife Agnes (middle), and Charlotte (right) while we vacationed together in St. Anton, Austria in 1970.

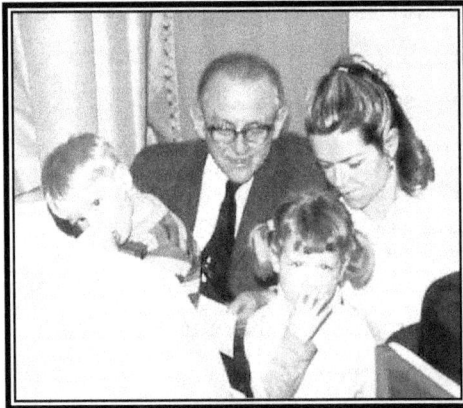

Figure 46. I took this photograph of Paul, my father, Charlotte, and Cheryl when we were visiting Vienna in 1972. The trip served as my family's first reunion with my parents following my departure from Hungary in 1956.

Unfortunately, Charlotte's gold bracelet was stolen from our hotel room in Vienna. We only realized the bracelet had been stolen when we returned home.

From then on, we visited Hungary, initially worrying about the admission permit to the country. Early in 1970, while we were waiting in the line at the Budapest airport passport check with the children, an AVO soldier with a machine gun suddenly approached us directly. I can remember thinking, "Oh boy! Now what?" Luckily for us, the soldier saw that our children were exhausted from the transatlantic flight; he escorted us to the front of the line so that we could clear customs without waiting. "How considerate," I thought.

On several occasions when we traveled to Hungary, we visited Budapest, Buda, the Castle Hill, Pécs and its surroundings, and the cottage in Badacsony. The political situation was getting better, but somehow it was always "tongue in cheek" with me. My bad dreams about the past regularly returned to haunt me.

In April 1974, my father attended the International Congress of Obstetrics and Gynecology Conference in New York City. We decided to drive to New York City to see him. Sure enough, on the way, in the Utica, New York, area, we drove into a blizzard and had to seek refuge overnight in a motel. Continuing to drive on the New York State Thruway was impossible until the weather and travel conditions improved!

On the occasion when I became a Fellow of the American College of Chest Physicians in San Francisco, California, we took my father, who was visiting us in the States, to the West Coast. It was quite a trip—trying to adjust my father to the time change, driving to Los Angeles on the Cabrillo Highway, visiting Hearst Castle and the Daniel family in Santa Barbara. My father became totally exhausted. Upon our return, he was delighted to see my home "West Oakfield," on Grand Island, New York.

My father's trip to the United States, this time, had not been without its emotional "ups and downs." As a matter of fact, it was tumultuous for him! Upon his arrival to the States, he lost his luggage full of Nikotas Munkás cigarette packs. He could not accept this loss and while returning to Hungary, he requested to see the Baggage "Lost and Found" at New York's Kennedy Airport. Of course, this area was so huge that he got lost in its "jungle." Not surprisingly, my father never found his suitcase there and began to accept the fact that its contents would have to be written off! Miraculously, two months later, the airlines delivered his suitcase to our home on Grand Island totally intact and full of my father's cigarettes!

My father received a letter at the end of 1974, advising him to retire and vacate his hospital apartment by June 30, 1975. Early in 1975, he acquired chickenpox for the second time, this time from one of his grandchildren. A few weeks later, he developed "Herpes Totalis" from his head to his feet. He was gravely ill. At that time, there was not any treatment for the herpes virus, except IV immune Ag A and B, which I obtained from Vienna and carried with me when I flew to Hungary. Hospitalized in the Dermatology wing of the University of Pècs Medical Center, my father was being treated by the professor of dermatology and Professor Hamori of the Internal Medicine Department.

While my father was getting over this tremendous illness, he got out of the bed one night to go to the bathroom, fell, and broke his vertebra. The chest x-ray showed a right upper lobe (RUL) peripheral lung nodule. The experts immediately established the diagnosis: carcinoma of the lung with metastasis to the spine. For the spine injury my father sustained, my father's doctors immobilized him in a "Plaster of Paris" bed. I suppose he was put on long-term cortisone as well because of the Herpes.

One night, he suffered massive gastrointestinal bleeding. They did a tracheostomy on him, and when he developed hypotension, they declared he also had a massive myocardial infarction. Shortly after he died, an autopsy was performed on him because by law in Hungary, "anybody who dies in the hospital has to have an autopsy." Thank God for this autopsy! The autopsy showed that my father did not have lung cancer. The lesion in the lung was a fungus ball, likely due to the prolonged cortisone treatment. His fractured vertebra was due to trauma, and he did not have coronary artery disease. The experts had gotten the diagnosis completely wrong.

In modern terms, he died of "immunological deficiency syndrome"— we may never be sure from what, but we definitely can make some reasonable assumptions. He was immunologically vulnerable when he acquired chickenpox the second time in his life; acquiring Herpes Totalis, he became an immunological cripple!

He died when he was seventy-one years of age, smoked at times one hundred cigarettes (Nicotex Munkás brand) a day, and had no evidence of lung cancer or coronary artery disease.

Medical professionals should study further this type of patient and his/her lifestyle. Under the circumstances, why did my father not develop either lung cancer or coronary artery disease during his lifetime?

My father was given a university funeral in accordance with "communist traditions." The family followed it with a Roman Catholic funeral conducted in secret. For these rites, I did not go home to Hungary, because I did not want to be part of the university "celebrations."

Instead, I spent Christmas 1975 with my mother in our "old" flat in the wing of the hospital, where my parents had lived since my father had become the chief of obstetrics and gynecology at the University of Pècs. It was a somber holiday due to the facts that my father recently had died, and it was our last Christmas in the flat in which our family had lived for close to thirty years. My mother had to move to a two-bedroom apartment, in a building built by the government, like many apartment buildings at that time.

My mother was in good shape at seventy-one years of age. She traveled to Egypt and went on other trips. We traveled to Hungary to visit her several times. Age gradually started to impact her health. She had difficulties walking into town to run her errands and going to the hairdresser once a week. She required a pacemaker, and later it had to be replaced. I checked the pacemaker every time I went to Hungary. She employed a woman who came to her apartment daily to care for her. She was hospitalized a few times. She broke her hip, which required surgery, and then this surgery had to be redone due to "poor" work. During one of my return visits, when she just was discharged from the hospital, she was having abdominal pain. I diagnosed acute gall bladder. I telephoned the doctor to readmit her and do a cholecystectomy. My mother sailed through this operation.

One day, my sister telephoned me to inform me that my mother had a lump on her breast. She underwent a lumpectomy; the malignant tumor was not metastatic. Why does a ninety-four year old woman develop breast cancer? This certainly is a medical enigma. By now, my mother could hardly walk. She had had her wedding ring stolen from her, while she was in the hospital, and most of her jewelry was stolen from her flat by the different housemaids. She still was mentally sharp. When I saw her in March 1996, she asked me to get her a walker, so she could start to try to walk again. One month later, in April 1996, she died in her sleep, while her maid was doing food shopping. I do not think her death was caused by failure of her pacemaker, which I checked in March when I visited her. She had a very special funeral in a church, by now, with many of her and our friends attending. My nephew Tamas appeared at his grandmother's funeral church service in jeans; it's hard to forgive him for dressing this way on this sad occasion.

Shortly after my mother's death, my sister, my brother, and I gathered at my mother's flat, where we divided equally my mother's and parents' personal property, which included paintings, silver, etc. I resigned my rights (i. e. one-third) to the cottage at Badacsony, one of my best decisions in a long time.

As I have named it and will explain, the "curse of Badacsony," continued with a fierce battle between my sister's and my brother's families and my brother's son, Tamas. Finally, my sister Judy withdrew from the deal; she received very small compensation for her half of the cottage and property! The paradox of the matter was that the cottage needed to be completely renovated—it had been deteriorating since my father's death. The only person who could pay for these renovations was Tamas. After the Second World War, my father had been the only person who could save the cottage from the communists. Because both deals created huge family fights, I refer to the circumstances as the "curse of Badascony!"

After Tamas acquired the cottage, I went back more than once to sail on Lake Balaton at Balatonfüred. The first time I went with my English friends to the Kisfaludy Ház (a restaurant) in Badacsony, we did not stop to see the cottage; we were not invited! The second time, in 2005, Tamas was more gracious and invited us with my Scottish friends, the Orrs. The cottage is beautiful—it is nicely reconstructed with terracing. The water runoff is channeled away from the house. Its three floors are livable, with air conditioning and heating. On the lowest level, there is a garage. Now the cottage often serves as a relaxing retreat for Tamas and his family and, less frequently, for my brother. My brother and Agnes like to stay there when nobody else is there.

Charlotte refused to go and see the newly renovated cottage. My sister periodically vacations in Badacsony, but she also refuses to visit the cottage! The "curse" of Badacsony still lingers, and I only hope it will not continue to haunt Tamas's and Ivan's children! Certainly, many "hard" feelings about the cottage and the deals involving it still remain.

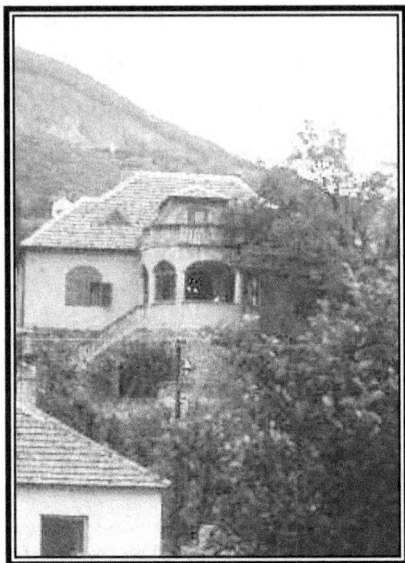

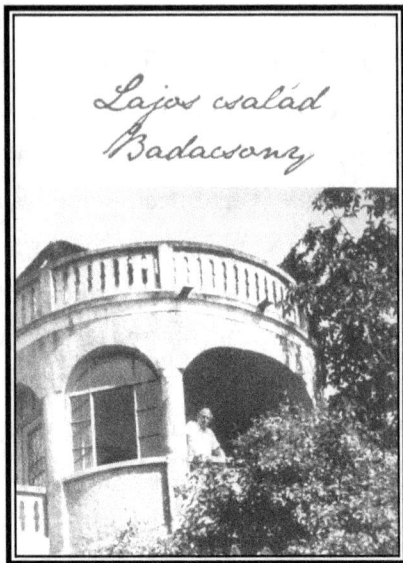

Figures 47-48. Left: The cottage at Badacsony, Hungary. Right: My Father is enjoying the view from the open porch. The family cottage is located on the slopes of Badascony Mountain, where basalt rock once was excavated. Now excavations are against the law.

PART III
THE PROFESSIONAL YEARS:
TRAINING IN GENERAL SURGERY

GENERAL SURGICAL TRAINING IN THE GALLIE COURSE, UNIVERSITY OF TORONTO, ONTARIO, CANADA: 1961-1963

After my one-year fellowship at the Banting Institute ended in July 1961, I was accepted provisionally into the Gallie training course in general surgery.

My first half-year assignment at the University of Toronto was as a first year surgical resident on cardiovascular surgery.

The teaching of residents was organized very well. The residents' responsibilities were clear: rounds were conducted weekly, and we had to present the cases. Incidentally, we were given the responsibility of presenting three types of cases: interesting cases, problematic cases, and rare cases. The residents presented the first type of case; the chief resident, the second; and fellows, the third. Drs. Gordon Thomas and Wolf Saperstein were spending an extra year following the completion of their training to help out with the more difficult cases.

Four attending physicians served on staff: Dr. Wilfred Bigelow, Chief of

Cardiovascular Surgery, Dr. Jim Key, Dr. Ray Heimbecker, and the newest member, having just arrived home from his McLaughlin Traveling Fellowship in Russia, Dr. Ronald Baird. Dr. Baird felt that his professional time had been wasted in Russia. Previously, Drs. W. Bigelow, H. Swan, and M. DeBakey were invited on advisory travel trips to the Soviet Union to establish and maintain an ongoing connection with Russian cardiac surgeons. With the exception of Dr. Bigelow's report, which was benign, Dr. Swan's and Dr. DeBakey's described and then evaluated the poor and primitive state of Russian cardiac surgery.

Dr. Robert Ginsburg was my fellow house officer, while I completed the cardiac surgery rotation. We became good friends and remained so for many years. Bob specialized in thoracic surgery and then proceeded to become the chief of thoracic surgery at Memorial Sloan-Kettering Cancer Center in New York City. After a few years, he returned to Toronto, where in later years, he became the chief of thoracic surgery at the University of Toronto. Unfortunately, a heavy smoker during his life, Bob died from carcinoma of the lung.

Open-heart cases were "big cases" at that time requiring full operating room mobilization. The cases such as the ones involving the removal of steel shrapnel from the heart of an eleven-year-old boy, the artificially "hibernated kid," and an adult with retroperitoneal seminoma could never be forgotten. By that time, Peter Kuypers had left the program and Peter Blundell became the chief resident of cardiovascular surgery. One day while assisting Dr. Blundell with the removal of the shrapnel from the heart of the young boy, Dr. Blundell made a sly remark: "Nowadays we have to operate with a team of physicians originating from many different countries."

The second assistant also was a Hungarian doctor escapee like me. Dr. Peter Blundell was a "funny" guy, born into the Torontonian "high society." Even after many years living among these people, he seemed to be jealous. "How do you end up with the most fashionable girls all the time?" he asked me a few years later.

Dr. W. Bigelow, Uncle Bill as he was known, was a charming individual with strong beliefs and determinations; he possessed and used his excellent political skills. He emerged victorious from the battle with his senior, Dr. Gordon Murray, for the chair of cardiovascular surgery. G. Murray was a superb surgeon and researcher; he possessed many cutting-edge, new, and extremely innovative ideas. Murray was more paranoid than shy, while Bigelow was more didactic, a better teacher, less of a surgeon, and the slier politician. My relationship with Dr. Bigelow is described well in the Festschrift reprinted below in Appendix 6.

Some of Dr. Bigelow's remarks in the operating room were "everlasting." One day, when a "bad" patient having surgery was not doing well, Uncle Bill asked the anesthetist how much oxygen he was giving to the patient, "100% O2," the anesthetist replied. Dr. B. said sternly: "You have to give more than 100% in these cases."

Another day the patient did not defibrillate to restart the heart after the repair. While the patient was still on the pump, Dr. B tried to get the patient to defibrillate by means of the defibrillator at least ten times without success. Finally, he said: "Please turn the lights off; they are draining too much electricity." He always became very serious and hard on himself when the patient did not do well.

There were three steady and excellent anesthesiologists on staff. One day, a patient died during an operation from a massive air embolism through the radial line. The anesthesiologist had to talk to the patient's relatives. He ended up leaving the Toronto General Hospital shortly afterwards.

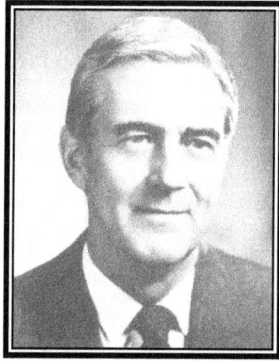

Figures 49-50. Pictured here are Dr. Bigelow (top) and (bottom) Drs. Heimbecker, Baird, Bigelow, and Key.

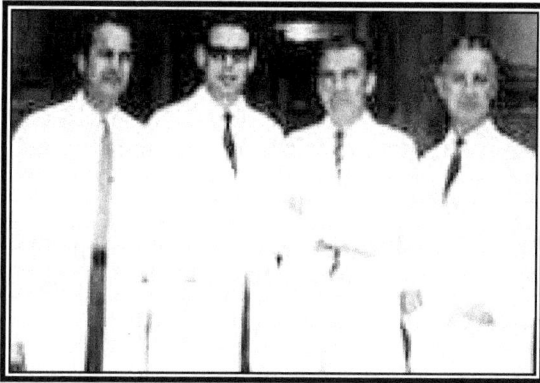

Dr. Bigelow assigned me to a project that turned out to be quite interesting. Because Dr. Bigelow always believed that the Vineberg pedicle worked, he kept performing this type of operation. Consequently, I had to take his patients to the cardiology department and connect them to eleven electrical wires to record the EKG at rest, during walking, and afterwards. The results were equivocal. At that time, even the two- step Master's test was unknown. I should have developed a standard protocol

181

at that time for the stress EKGs. Dr. Bigelow decided to send one of his patients to the Cleveland Clinic, to Dr. Mason Sones, who selectively catheterized the patient's mammary artery and definitely showed collateralization of the pedicle with the coronary arteries. How much? Was it enough? These questions remained unanswered for a while and became an extensive research topic many years later!

Heparin was used most of the time for induction of cardiopulmonary bypass, prevention of thrombosis in bypass grafts on the lower extremities, and for pulmonary embolisms. Dr. W. Bigelow described it in detail in his book, titled *Mysterious Heparin, The Key to Open Heart Surgery.* Heparin was discovered by Dr. Jay McLean, when McLean was working as a research assistant at Johns Hopkins during the 1920s. As Dr. Bigelow accurately described, Dr. McLean had a sad career and never received the acknowledgment that he deserved. Heparin was produced first by Cannaught Laboratories in Toronto and was first surgically applied probably in the 1930s by Dr. Gordon Murray, while he was performing a saphenous vein bypass on a patient following the removal of a popliteal aneurysm.

We residents were involved in the application of Heparin in certain situations such as those involving pulmonary embolisms, acute arterial thrombosis of the lower extremities, and peripheral arterial embolization. During Dr. Murray's time, the Heparin dosage was determined by counting the IV fluid drops from the Heparin bottle. Because the operating room nurses complained to Dr. Murray that they were unable to constantly watch and count the drops, Dr. Murray then set up a system of light beams interrupted by the drops. This system enabled the number of drops to be registered and counted simultaneously at the nursing station. In our time, the drips and IVs already were standardized, but we had to determine the clotting times every four hours and calculate the dosages from them; this oftentimes necessitated performing clotting time analyses throughout the night, every four hours.

At the conclusion of open-heart surgery, one-to-one Polybren was given, because we did not know exactly the required balance. Postoperative bleeding frequently occurred, so Polybren was removed from the drug market because of its side effects. Protamine is given nowadays in a one-to-one ratio, and clotting times and circulating Heparin are measured with different blood viscosity analyzers (ex. Sono-Clot measuring the blood viscosity).

My previous mentor in the lab at the Banting Institute, Dr. Raymond Heimbecker, was a very active member of the team. He always was "dreaming" about a new procedure and innovations in the operative protocol. In 1961, he decided to do a mitral valve replacement with a homologous aortic valve on a patient. (This was one of the experiments I had conducted the previous year at the Banting Institute.) The patient lived for five to seven days. The patient's heart disease was too far advanced, and he had Stage IV heart failure. Hemodynamically, the valve worked ok.

Ray always was available in cases of any emergency. "If things are gray, call Ray," we used to say. However, the challenge for us oftentimes involved finding him. Sometimes he could be found sleeping on a couch in a side room. Upon rising, he used to say, "I am racing against time," and he would take care of the problem at hand. On his list of hobbies, he included sailing and and remote-controlled, model airplanes and motor boats. He reported four cases of surgically-treated resection of acute myocardial infarction at the meeting of the Society of University Surgeons.

Ray became the chief of cardiovascular surgery in London, Ontario, Canada. Very early in the game, he became involved in cardiac transplantation, using Cyclosporine. His home always was open to me; there I met his charming wife and his children. It was devoid of hypocrisy or snobbery; Ray and his family were very down-to-earth and humble.

Ray decided to buy old logs, which he collected from old Canadian log cabins; he screened the wood and built a beautiful log cabin for his family in the Muskoka region of Ontario, Canada; there he undoubtedly had the chance to play with his remote-controlled airplanes and motor boats.

The youngest staff member, Dr. Ronald Baird, was the rising star. He possessed a brilliant mind, was a Rhodes Scholar as well as a great surgeon and person. He always was a tremendous help to me. We published together several papers, and later I sailed with his son Ron on my boat. When Dr. Bigelow retired, Ron became the chief for ten years. He refused his second term of ten years. Fern, his wife, told me, he later experienced periods of depression.

My half-year on the cardiac service passed in no time. As usual, before our next assignments, we were required to meet with Chairman of the Department of Surgery Dr. Frederick Kergin. He always carefully evaluated us based upon the half-year report from the last service in the different surgery divisions. In general, he was satisfied with my work, but he told me then and each time in the future during which I met with him: "We are going to train you, but why don't you go back home afterwards?" He did not seem to understand that I could not go back home to Hungary, a communist country I had fled. Without success, I tried to explain the situation to him, but he continued to suggest that I should return to Hungary.

Around this time, in the early 1960s, I received a letter from my father stating that he was planning to go to Vienna, Austria, to attend a meeting there. Since my vacation was imminent, I arranged my affairs so that I could go to Europe to meet my parents in Vienna. A couple of days before my planned departure, I received a letter from England, demanding that I advance a certain amount of money for my stay there in 1957. Because I could not afford both, to fulfill the bill and the cost of my trip to Vienna, I was forced to cancel my trip overseas. Because of an ongoing family feud, I did not disclose to my parents the real reason for cancelling my trip. Stupidly, I sent them a telegram stating that I was cancelling my trip, because I became sick with Subacute Bacterial Endocarditis (SBE). My parents despaired at the news, and I had a hard time convincing them that everything was ok and that they should not worry about me.

For the next half-year surgery rotation, I was sent to Division II Surgery, where Dr. Mills served as chief and his attending surgeons included Drs. Robert Mustard and J. Palmer. This was a challenging assignment! I mostly worked with Mustard and Palmer, while Mills's resident was Dr. Ernie Sterns, senior house officer, who later served as an attending physician at the Kingston General Hospital of Queen's University. While Palmer was an easygoing, head and neck and plastic surgeon, Mustard was the opposite. He was obsessive, demanding, humorless, and apparently not very interested in the well-being of surgical fellows. He admitted his patients the night before their surgeries, and we were required to know everything about them the day before surgery so we could warn Mustard if problems existed or were foreseeable. I never had a half-day off from work for six months. I had an on-call room on the first floor of the private patient pavilion and shared this room with Dr. Claude LaBrosse, who had his own apartment and already had been accepted into the cardiac training program, which he would begin a few years later.

I learned meticulous, fine, and excellent surgery from both Palmer and Mustard, but Mustard only let me cut his patients' sutures. He never turned over his patients' surgeries or parts of them to me for teaching purposes. Palmer was more generous when it came to teaching surgical residents like me.

Every month, this division had grand rounds with Professor Kergin.

One time, Kergin openly drew the attention of the whole division to the fact that I managed to put up one cervical spine film upside down on the view light box. Kergin corrected the placement of the film himself. Anyway, as a whole this rotation became a very useful and rewarding one for me. As a senior resident, Dr. Ernie Sterns was a great help; he was very didactic, but I also learnt a lot from him.

One of the highlights of my training process was Dr. Tovie's Sunday 8:00 a.m. rounds of Division-I patients (i.e. Dr. Tovie's Sunday "mass"). These two hours were the quintessence of learning. Dr. Tovie's residents were assigned the task of presenting these patients' cases; from that point onward, he analyzed their histories, physical workups, and laboratory tests. He asked us individually what we would do for each patient. These sessions yielded ample constructive criticism from Dr. Tovie. If one was incorrect in how one would manage the patient's case, then Tovie would say: "You failed!" But his approach to evaluating us was never offensive!

We enjoyed only a few parties during my one-and-a-half year residency at the Toronto General Hospital, but by and large, we did not have enough time for partying and socializing. During one of these parties, I got to know Arthur Carman, the Greek who participated a few times. He was a great lover of pretty women. Later he established the best steakhouse in Toronto: Carman's Dining Club. This restaurant stayed in business until the mid-2000s. Carman also organized the yearly, international Toronto folk festival. At another one of these parties, the fellows got slightly drunk and decided to throw the antiquated television set out of the window. Many times previously a newer unit had been requested, to no avail. However, when this time it fell on a car in the doctors' parking lot, shortly afterwards a brand new television appeared in the residents' recreation room.

My next six-month assignment luckily was on the gynecological service in the General Hospital. Having grown up with a father who was an accomplished chief of gynecology and obstetrics at the University of Pècs, I really did not need this rotation since I already had learned so much from my father. I had a good working relationship with Dr. Manny Spivak, the chief resident on the service, and I found Dr. Canal to be nice, fair, friendly, and well-respected. Many patients on this service were drug addicts and prostitutes; operative gynecology was scarce. Only moderate numbers of these surgeries were performed.

By this time, my father had managed to contact Professor Canal, who gave him a good report on my performance. This report made the atmosphere less stressful, and I finished the service with good marks.

My next rotation was in urology at Sunnybrook Hospital. This rotation became extremely important. I submitted my application to write the Fellow of the Royal College of Surgeons Canada (i.e. the FRCS(C)) Exam in September, and if I passed it, I would have to take the oral exam in November. I spent the next six months studying, but I also had time for a few pleasures, since this service was not extremely busy.

The urology service was very well organized by Dr. Ian Todd, the chief resident. Incidentally, Ian was the first one in Canada who transplanted a kidney. A good surgeon, he was very smart, pleasant, and efficient. During my time completing this rotation, I assisted Dr. Robertson, another urologist, a few times. During one surgery he did a radical nephrectomy for renal cell carcinoma. At that time, I never predicted that one day I would do a case in which we had to place the patient on the heart-lung bypass in order to ream out his inferior vena cava (IVC) and remove a metastasized right atrial tumor, while simultaneously the urologist also performed surgery. This was the seventh reported case in the literature in 1987. Today this operation is routinely done for palliation.

Every other weekend, I was off duty. During the winter when I was off duty, I made frequent trips to the east—to the Lake Placid, Stowe, and

Sugarbush ski resorts—to go skiing with friends. These weekend getaways became a "habit" for us. By that time, I'd managed to sell my old Chevy and had bought a new Austin Healey Sprite. While it had excellent mileage, it did not have any spare room, certainly not for skis! How I was able to afford this car I do not know!

The surgical course at the University of Toronto was run in accordance with great organization, strict rules, and severe discipline when it was merited. Take, for example, the case of my fellow house officer, who was called one morning at 4:00 a.m. and told that one of the patients was distended, had overflow incontinence, and was in a miserable state. He shrugged off the patient's predicament and responded, "I will be in the hospital anyway at 7:00 a.m. and will catheterize the patient then." Learning about the delay, the chief of urology telephoned the orderly to instruct him to immediately do the catheterization. The chief of urology fired my fellow trainee in the morning. Later, this same doctor was dismissed from the surgical course.

Time passed quickly for me on the urology service, and since it was well organized, I also found time to study. I kept in contact with Marv Tile and his family. Marv and I frequently discussed and examined various surgery topics.

Professor Kergin met with me after the half-year evaluation, and as usual, told me he would train me, but recommended that I go home to Hungary afterwards. I always responded, "I cannot go back to Hungary." He mentioned the available chief residency positions at Sunnybrook Hospital, Wellesley Hospital, and the Toronto General Hospital. I told him I preferred the position at Toronto General. By now, I had become more outspoken. Kergin asked me, "Why?"

"Because it is the best!" I responded.

"What about Sunnybrook?" he asked me.

"I do not want it, but I will take any position you will give me, Sir," said. I left Kergin's office after these discussions, and he did not elaborate further on the matter.

While I did not know where I would be working, I knew I would be able to take at least two weeks off to study before I would have to start my new position as a chief resident. I was lucky Kergin assigned me to the Wellesley Hospital, which had a good reputation.

This was the time I managed to arrange for my mother to leave Hungary to visit me on a trip to Canada and decided that during her stay, we would rent a cottage in Algonquin Park for two weeks or possibly longer. My mother managed to get permission from the communist authorities to visit me in Canada. Per the communist protocol, I was required to guarantee that all her expenses would be paid for her; I sent a letter stating that I would fulfill this obligation. My mother came to Canada in June 1963 and lived in Toronto in a rented room close to the Wellesley Hospital. During the period when I was changing my job assignments, we went to the cottage close to Algonquin Park. There I studied all day and swam twice a day, while my mother enjoyed the surroundings and cooked for me. We had the best time together, while I tried my utmost to prepare for my written examination.

CHIEF RESIDENT AT THE WELLESLEY HOSPITAL, TORONTO, ONTARIO, CANADA: JULY 1963- JULY 1964

⌒≋⌒

The Wellesley Hospital was quite a place in the summer of 1963. Dr. Ian McDonald was the chief of the surgery service. Drs. Robert Mitchell, Ted Mullens, and Neal Waters served as his associates. Of course, as the most junior member of the team, I more or less worked as Dr. McDonald's slave, but luckily not for too long. McDonald was a fussy, average general surgeon, who knew everything that was happening in surgery and in the hospital, since he had a close relationship with the operating room supervisor Ms. DeRose.

Dr. R. Mitchell, an Australian, had passed five examinations for Royal College of Surgeons' fellowships (FRCS). He did all the chest cases and some general surgery ones. He was married into the Watson family, the same family that owned several supermarket chains in North America and the United Kingdom. Mitchell certainly did not lack money!

Dr. T. Mullens was the youngest and was a good, all-around general surgeon. He was pleasant and witty.

Dr. Neal Waters was the most senior in ranking and age after Dr. McDonald. He was very particular, precise, meticulous, and quite prone to splitting hairs at times but still managed to do good surgery.

At the end of the summer, all hell broke loose! While I was assisting Dr. McDonald in July, Dr. McDonald stopped for a second and told me: "I will go for a holiday in August. Dr. Waters will be in charge until I return." He never returned! Leaving his wife and family, he moved to San Francisco, took his bank accounts etc. with him, and married the heiress to the Avis Rent a Car fortune. Nobody, including his family, knew this bomb was coming beforehand. They undoubtedly were as devastated as we were surprised!

From then on, I worked with the other three surgeons, running a busy service, and at times covered urology too. In early September 1963, I wrote the first part of my fellowship examination. The questions required essay answers. For example, one of them asked, "What do you know about the tricuspid valve?" Shortly after writing the examination, before I had gotten my examination results, I had a routine appointment with Dr. Kergin. The meeting was going fine until I told him that I was taking my FRCS examination. He then declared: "You will fail. Do not take it this year!" At that point, I felt I could not withdraw from the examination, so I told him I would rather take the chance than lose the money I paid to register for and take the exam. A month later, in October, I was informed that I passed part one and would be notified when my oral exam was scheduled in Montreal for some time in November 1963! Following this news, I began to study hard for part two. In preparation, I studied with Marv Tile and Ernie Sterns, who quizzed me, and I attended Dr. Tovie's patient rounds on Sunday mornings.

The Wellesley Hospital Surgical Service was good and quite pleasant without Dr. McDonald. One of the chest surgeons came over from

Toronto Western Hospital to do thoracoabdominal esophagectomies. Dr. L. was very good, slick, and fast—he could do the surgery in less than two hours—but every gastro-esophageal anastomosis he did leaked. Some of his patients survived, while some died. Waters's anastomoses were better but were very lengthy surgeries.

My big exam date in November was fast approaching! At this time, I committed another blunder with my family, but I was lucky, and in the end, I achieved one of the greatest successes of my life.

The date was set for my oral exam—if I remember well, it was scheduled for a Friday in November 1963. Since I practically had no time off from work to finish getting prepared, I planned to fly to Montreal on Thursday, take the exam on Friday, and fly back to Toronto on the same day on the late, direct flight. I informed my parents about the dates and timing for my trip.

The undeniable success was that I passed the oral examination of the Royal College of Surgeons of Canada, F.R.C.S.(C). One of my examiners happened to be the "dreaded" head and neck surgeon, the chairman of the department of surgery at the University of Saskatchewan in Saskatoon, a New Zealander. He was well-known as the toughest and most rigorous examiner. This expert mostly asked head and neck questions. Thank God, my exam went smoothly. I was elated and very happy! I decided to drive home to Toronto, after I secured a refund for half of my trip's airfare.

The weather turned bad after 4:00 p. m., when the rain came down in buckets. Heading home, I drove past Montréal–Dorval International Airport about the time my plane was supposed to depart for Toronto. One hour later, I heard the terrible news on my car radio. The exact airplane on which I had been scheduled to return to Toronto crashed shortly after takeoff and all passengers died. I thanked God for my good luck!

I drove home to Toronto and went to work the next morning. Upon leaving the operating room after a case, I was told that a long distance telephone call was waiting for me. My father had been listening to the BBC broadcast as he always did, when he heard that the plane I was supposed to take home to Toronto the previous day had crashed. It took a short time to convince my parents that I was ok and that I had passed the oral examination, but they were not very happy that I had not let them know I'd decided to drive back to Toronto from Montreal. C'est la vie!

When the news that I passed the oral examination began to circulate, the attending surgeons were happy; they began to give me a share in their operating room work. Shortly afterwards, I had another "check-up" session with Professor Kergin. What a tremendous change in his behavior as he received me! He stood up and warmly shook my hand, congratulating me for my success. He asked his secretary to bring me a cup of tea or coffee, and finally we had a warm discussion together. He offered to get me a position in the department of thoracic surgery at the Royal Brompton Hospital in London, UK. He was pleased to hear that Dr. Heimbecker had secured a job for me with Dr. C. Rollins Hanlon in St. Louis, Missouri, U.S.A.

The ceremony for the conferral of the FRCS certificates (i.e. graduation into the "club") was scheduled for the January meeting of the Royal College of Surgeons of Canada in Quebec City, Canada. The snow at that time was perfect for skiing. The day before graduation, I went skiing with some of my colleagues who also were receiving their certificates. Dr. Dave Hastings was with us. An excellent skier, Dave had the misfortune of falling in the woods and seeming to break his neck. Fortunately, Dr. Tom Barrington was with him when this accident occurred. When the emergency rescue team placed Dave on the sleigh to be skied down to the bottom of the slopes, Tom supervised Dave's care. Kneeling on the sleigh, Tom kept Dave's head in between his knees as Dave was skied down to the bottom of the slopes and hospitalized. Fortunately, he had some neurological signs only in his arms, which disappeared after the emergency fusion.

On November 22, 1963, President Kennedy was assassinated in Dallas, Texas. I was driving in heavy rain on Jarvis Street in Toronto when I heard the news. Totally stunned, I accidentally bumped the car ahead of me; luckily there was not any damage!

Christmas was approaching and the Wellesley Hospital was nicely decorated. The various floor units were having parties, and the atmosphere reminded me somewhat of that in Vienna when I had crossed the Iron Curtain from Hungary into Austria in December 1956 and lodged in Vienna for the holiday season. During the holidays of 1963, I got to know better Charlotte Scott, my future wife.

I have written about our story elsewhere, but I will recount a shorter version of it here. An emergency room nurse who worked at Wellesley Hospital, Charlotte was the girlfriend of my friend and roommate at the Toronto General Hospital, Dr. Claude LaBrosse. Our relationship became an ongoing, developing one. After she finished work in the evening, we would on occasion eat dinner together. Since she liked Chinese food, we went to Sai Woo's (Sai Woo Garden Restaurant) in Toronto's Chinatown. After a few dinners there, I realized that on the floor just above our heads, every Wednesday, a meeting of some sort was occurring. The meeting turned out to be the regular meeting of the Canadian Communist Party. At that time, the communist party still had Canadian support.

Around this time my pediatric professor from medical school, Dr. Kerpel-Fronius, visited The Hospital for Sick Children of the University of Toronto. His daughter Eva traveled from Boston, where she was attending college, to see her father. We were invited to Dr. Sass-Kortsak's home. Sass-Kortsak was the "Wilson disease" expert at the Hospital for

Sick Children. He was a balloon head, a conceited egotist, and was not nice at all. One day, I drove the Kerpels up to Algonquin Park and showed them the lake district—we had a pleasant trip. When I was in Boston, I stayed with Professor Gamble, Kerpel's previous tutor, who did basic research on small children's nutritional states and electrolytes. Gamble's beautiful house was situated in the Boston suburb of Brookline Village.

One day I was called out of the operating room to talk to the Royal Canadian Mounted Police (RCMP), who were waiting for me downstairs. "Where are the skis you bought in Stowe, Vermont, at such and such a time?" they inquired. I told them that they were stored in the basement of my friend's house. They wanted me to retrieve them since they were confiscating them; I had not declared them at Customs and consequently had not paid the Canadian Customs duty on them when I entered Canada with them after I bought them in the U.S.A. The police told me that the only thing I could do to reclaim my personal property was to go to the auction and buy them back. Of course, I did not have any time to go to the auction at its given time. I lost my new skis to the police in spite of what seemed like a legitimate defense to me—because I broke my old skis and had to buy a new pair.

I tried to convince the police that I had not done anything wrong by drawing an analogy—I told them that when I blew a tire while driving in the U.S., I had to buy a new one to get home. All these arguments were in vain! The RCMP likely went to the ski shops in the U.S., where they obtained a list of Canadian buyers from the manufacturers. They checked who paid or did not pay duty on the merchandise.

A similar situation had arisen a couple of years before when I drove from Detroit, Michigan, to Newport Beach, California. I camped during this car trip in my pup tent. I drove through Telluride, Colorado, the Four Corners, and the Navajo reservation. I spent a day at the south rim of the

Grand Canyon, where I met two Canadian high school graduates, with whom I descended into the Canyon to the Colorado River, where we spent a couple of hours swimming and eating. After 2:00 p.m., we started to hike back up to the top of the south rim. It became harder and harder to get back to the top; we took more frequent rests in the over-100-degree Fahrenheit sunshine. One of the men declared that he would not be able to make the hike to the rim top; he decided to sleep or rest for a couple of hours. The other chap and I made it to the top before sunset, and by midnight, the second one also had hiked to the rim top. Luckily he made it, because the temperatures had plummeted to forty degrees Fahrenheit after nightfall!

After delivering the car to Newport Beach, I traveled to San Francisco, where I visited a couple of nurses from Toronto East General Hospital. On the trip back east, while I was in the San Francisco airport, the airlines made me pay for my pup tent as an extra piece of luggage. Because I did not have any money, I had to borrow some from the nurses who had driven me to the airport. Upon arrival in Toronto, the pup tent was lost. I claimed it with the airline, and it gave me some money equivalent to the value of the tent. The next year when I needed a tent for another trip, I went to a pawnshop on Yonge Street in Toronto to buy a used one. Upstairs in the shop, I found my old pup tent, which I recognized since it included two bayonets I had purchased years ago to use in place of the regular aluminum pegs as stakes. The shopkeepers sold me my old tent for a smaller price than I had paid for it. You can believe that I said nothing about how I had lost the tent and how the airline had reimbursed me full price the previous year. I always have wondered how the shop possessed my tent, but so far, I have not solved this mystery!

Around this time, my mentor Professor Donhoffer also visited Toronto, for some reason I do not remember. I was thrilled to take him around the city for one day, to introduce him to my future wife Charlotte, and to have a delicious steak dinner at Carman's. By that time, I had an open account at Carman's. A few weeks before, I experienced a great evening at Carman's with Charlotte. When it came time to pay on this former occasion, I realized that I had left my wallet at home and Charlotte also did not have any money with her. Carman was understanding and asked me to bring him the money for our dinner at my convenience. The next morning, on a Sunday at 8:00 a.m., when I appeared at his door, he opened the upstairs window of the restaurant and told me to slip the money under his front door. He must have had a great and rough night!

In the New Year, I submitted my request to the American government to immigrate to the U.S.A. and get a visa to work as a fellow on the cardiac surgery unit at St. Louis University Hospital, where I had my next appointment. The entry visa would not be issued until the end of June, because my name had to be placed on and taken from the list of waiting Hungarian immigrants. Because I was getting desperate, I went with Charlotte to meet with the U.S. Consul in Toronto about this matter. After orientation, he asked Charlotte about her nationality by birth and the fact that we planned to get married on June 27, 1964. When she disclosed that she had been born in Canada, the Consul declared, "No problem under the circumstances. Your husband will be issued an immigrant visa. Your marriage will enable him to get a visa and eliminate the need to grant him a visa from the list of Hungarians waiting to enter the country as part of the Hungarian quota!" Wow, that had worked!

On June 27, 1964, Charlotte and I married at the St. Clare Catholic Church on the corner of Dufferin and St. Clair Streets in Toronto. A few family members attended our nuptials. Due to the influence of my future father-in-law, Charlotte and I did not have to complete "prenuptial Catholic instruction." When it came time during the ceremony to put the simple gold wedding band on her finger, I could not find it in my pocket.

I had a hole in my pocket through which the ring got lost in the inner lining. After the ceremony, we went home to my in-laws' house, located at 96 King High Avenue, where we lunched with Charlotte's sister Catherine, her grandmother Great Nana, and her parents. From the house, we departed in my Austin Healey Sprite to our honeymoon in Montreal. When we returned to Toronto from the Laurentian Mountains on July 4, 1964, we loaded the back of my "roomy" car with our extra luggage and sped off in it to St. Louis, Missouri, where my future bosses anxiously awaited my arrival on my new job.

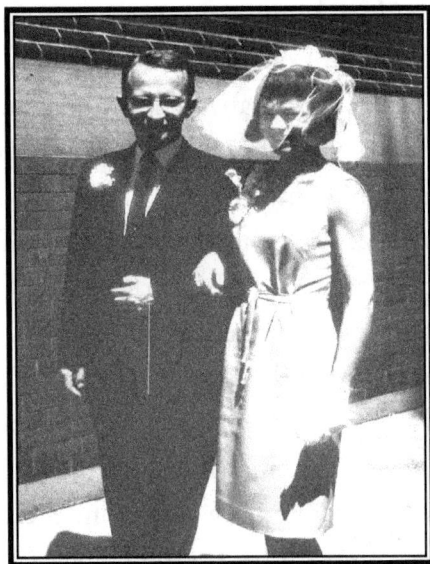

Figure 51. Just married! My lovely wife, Charlotte (maiden name: Scott), and I stand outside St. Clare Catholic Church in Toronto, Ontario, Canada, on our wedding day June 27, 1964.

Upon arrival in St. Louis, we did not have anywhere to stay, because we had not made any living arrangements. We roomed in a Diplomat Motel for three or four days, until we ran out of money. I started work the first day, while Charlotte unhappily was left alone. We secured a rental room with a shared bathroom on the third floor of a nearby house. That certainly was not the best solution, but we endured it for a few weeks, until we moved into a one-bedroom apartment. Because we did not have any furniture and could not afford any, we bought lawn furniture upon which we slept and sat. No doubt these were hard times in a strange city for newlyweds! In addition, I had to work every day, since I was the only fellow on the cardiac surgery unit.

Fully trained in Toronto, I used to say, "If I can get an academic job in Toronto in cardiac surgery, I will be willing to surrender ten years of my life." How stupid! "What is bad today may be good tomorrow, and what is good today may be bad tomorrow!" Circumstances do change, sometimes for the better and sometimes for the worse, but they inevitably do change. Change is almost certain, like taxes and death.

THOMAS Z. LAJOS

PART IV
THE PROFESSIONAL YEARS:
TRAINING IN CARDIAC AND
THORACIC SURGERY

200

FELLOW ON CARDIAC SURGERY SERVICE, ST. LOUIS UNIVERSITY MEDICAL CENTER: JULY 1964-JULY 1965

~⁂~

St. Louis University is managed and governed by the Jesuits in St. Louis, Missouri. The hospital was built by the Firmin Desloge family. It looks like an pancake. Flanked by rooms, a corridor extended down the middle of the building, which was ten to twelve stories high. For many years, it was the tallest building in St. Louis. Neighboring it, the SSM Cardinal Glennon Children's Medical Center was built later. These two hospitals were my territory of work.

Trained at Johns Hopkins University School of Medicine and one of Dr. Blalock's first residents, Dr. C. Rollins Hanlon was the chief of surgery at St. Louis University Medical Center. He came to St. Louis in the middle of the 1950s, became the chairman of the department of surgery, and started performing heart surgery. He made the service better, busier, and more famous than the one at Barnes-Jewish Hospital, which also is in St. Louis.

Dr. Hanlon was an exceptional individual; he was a stern, almost ascetic, devoted Catholic, who attended masses almost daily whenever he could. He was an excellent presenter; his English was impeccable, and his presentations were scholarly masterpieces delivered in the manner of a commanding chief. Daily he appeared in an ironed white coat, wearing a straw hat. He could be rather severe with the residents, but his focus always was concerned wholly with their educations and training; at all times, he concentrated on teaching the residents. In all aspects of his approach, he evinced the traditions of Johns Hopkins University School of Medicine. He was a meticulous surgeon—for example, he lost minimal amounts of blood while doing an adult coarctation, snapping all bleeding spots. His operations often took a long time, but he perfectly did his job in the tradition of William Stewart Halstead (1852-1922). The professor, Dr. Hanlon, always stayed with his patients, overnight if his patients were critical.

Once he gave the memorial lecture on Dr. Evarts Graham, describing Graham's surgical contributions (i.e. first pneumonectemy for cancer and contribution for empyema care) and depicting Graham as a very pleasant and kind individual, which he was not! In heart surgery, Washington University's Barnes-Jewish Hospital lagged behind St. Louis University Hospital, which was thriving. Dr. Graham was extremely hard on the residents, as was his successor, Dr. Thomas Burford. He could be brutal; his reputation was known nationwide.

Dr. Vallee Willman was second in command on this service; he trained in and graduated from St. Louis University's surgery program. A "milder" individual, easier to approach, he was a teacher of tremendous knowledge and reputation. He and Dr. Hanlon got along well, but there was never a doubt in anyone's mind who the boss was. Dr. Willman was a slicker, more daring surgeon, who also juggled research responsibilities with Dr. George Kaiser, the youngest attending physician, from Indianapolis, trained there by Dr. Schumacher. Kaiser also was a knowledgeable individual; he always was available and helpful, but was nervous at times and excitable. Every time I assisted him, he always managed to nick my hand. His only hobby was singing in of one of the Barbershop Singers groups.

A physiologist and the director of research, Dr. Theodore Cooper was the fourth member of this service. Later he would become the Assistant Secretary of Health in the U.S. Department of Health, Education, and Welfare in Washington, D.C. Brilliant, he was less practical!

The St. Louis University group intensively was involved in cardiac autotransplantations; it sought to determine, "What happens to the heart when it is completely detached from the circulation? In other words, what happens to the heart when it has been denervated and transplanted?" The St. Louis group had written extensively on this topic. They documented the adrenalin deprivations in the cells of the transplanted myocardium.

In the animal laboratory, I assisted with several transplants on dogs and was assigned to do complete cardiac denervations on cats without the help of bypass. The totally denervated heart functions as a transplanted one for six to eight weeks as the measured myocardial adrenalin concentration gradually recovers. This was true for the transplanted heart but not for the "fully" denervated heart. Later, it turned out to be characteristic of the human transplanted heart too. The St. Louis group travelled to Texas and experimented on monkeys as well. The group was ready for human heart transplants but lost momentum. Dr. Lower with Dr. Shumway at Stanford already had transplanted a heart into a dog that lived for over one year.

In the beginning, I was lost clinically. The system in Toronto was totally different from the one in St. Louis. In Toronto, all procedures and surgeries were outlined and systematically planned, whereas as part of the St. Louis group, I had to learn about the atmosphere, system, organization, habits, rules, and the surgeons' ways of thinking. This approach required time to master.

For instance, I scrubbed for the thoracic cases until Dr. Hanlon pulled me aside to tell me that I should not "take" cases from the general surgery chief resident. I told Dr. Hanlon, "Why did you not tell me this from the beginning? I certainly will obey the rules." I do not know who initiated this setback for me, either the general surgery chief resident because he needed the cases for his certification or Dr. Hanlon, who provided the residents' chest cases for board approval.

Hanlon did not have an approved thoracic training program at this time; the system was the same as it existed at Johns Hopkins School of Medicine. Again, "calling the shots" first should not have caused controversy. I started to become more possessive with the cardiac cases in the operating room and on the floor. My year at St. Louis University Medical Center was marked by spectacular cases and shocking losses. While Hanlon and Willman possessed strong, "inflexible" ideas, they always were straightforward about matters and implemented the rules like gentlemen.

Dr. Gerry Geisler, the general surgical resident at St. Louis, was from Dallas, Texas. He had been present in the operating room at Parkland Memorial Hospital in Dallas when U.S. President John F. Kennedy arrived there "dead." Gerry and his wife had had a baby. One day, leaving their infant in the car, they ran into a supermarket for some food. Unfortunately, when they returned to their vehicle, the infant was dead. What an unbelievable catastrophe for them! I met Dr. G. several years later. Although he was much younger than I was, he stopped practicing surgery because he suffered from severe diabetic peripheral neuropathy.

The cases at St. Louis University Medical Center were challenging and difficult. We performed some of the first cardiac operations ever done, without any previous backup or experience pertaining to how to do them.

Take for instance, the case of a young woman, upon whom we completed an aortic valve replacement with femoral arterial perfusion. This case went well and after the woman's skin was closed, the surgeon noted a mole on the left upper quadrant of her chest, which he excised uneventfully. Returning for follow up six to eight months later, this patient showed widespread distribution of "malignant" melanomas below her umbilicus. The recurrence of melanoma was unexplained at that location. Clinically, the moles as malignant melanoma were verified on the pathological sections.

Another patient was admitted to our care with third-degree heart block. We started intravenous adrenalin for marked bradycardia. The same intravenous perfusion partially was maintained before and after surgery with Isuprel. This patient kept on having runs of ventricular fibrillation. I sat by her bedside and defibrillated her about thirty times during the night. Eventually she was discharged from the hospital to go home; at that time, she thanked me for my services but asked that I not "shock" her "so many times" next time. Today we know that it is dangerous to give intravenous inotropes to the patients who have third-degree heart block.

A left thoracotomy was performed on a young patient with coarctation of the aorta. During the operation, bleeding from the patient's lung tissue necessitated a lobectomy, and then later a pneumonectomy. The patient never recovered; he died on the operating room table.

A patient with university affiliation had lung surgery for cancer. His recovery was protracted with moderate bleeding occurring postoperatively. Finally, I was told maybe five to seven days later, to pull the patient's chest tube. When I did this, the patient hemorrhaged; after exploration, he was lost.

The chest surgeon in the Hospital, Dr. Lucido, did a fair amount of private surgery. He used huge (i.e. one and a half inches in diameter) chest tubes that he obtained from the pump circuitry to try to prevent postoperative air leaks from his patients' lungs.

SSM Cardinal Glennon Children's Medical Center, a teaching hospital for St. Louis University School of Medicine had somewhat of a competitive relationship with Dr. Lewis, the pediatric surgeon who was not doing open heart surgeries on children. One day an Atrial Septal Defect (ASD) secundum was done on the pump, both Interior Vena Cava (IVC) and Superior Vena Cava (SVC) cannulated but both not snared yet. When the patient went on the pump, since there was a pressure difference between the two vena cavae, the air from the tube recirculated and went through the existing ASD to the left side. The patient ended up with irreversible brain damage and died.

Dr. John Schweiss was the best cardiac anesthesiologist. He was the first person I knew who used the telephone in the operating room; most of the time, he would use the telephone to arrange his stocks on the stock market, while he watched the patient with a "hawk's eye." We used to call him Dr. Scheiss! "Scheiss" is the German word for "shit."

Dr. Schweiss was a keen observer; he was brilliantly knowledgeable and possessed good judgment. He never gossiped about operating room matters and was tight-lipped.

One day, upon returning from Johns Hopkins, Dr. Hanlon stated laconically, "The Chief has died." Of course we knew to whom he was referring: Dr. A. Blalock. We did not have to ask any more questions.

There was a first- or second-year general surgical resident for whom I felt sorry. He was treated abominably, perhaps because of his language problems. I never doubted his performance. He was a Syrian doctor, Dr. Sami Kabani, with whom I became good friends. Several times, Charlotte and I invited him to our apartment for dinner.

Sami persevered. After St. Louis, he spent a couple of years training in Houston with Dr. D. Cooley and a year or two elsewhere; he developed a close professional relationship with Sir Donald Ross of Guy's Hospital, London. We remained good friends for years; I met him frequently at different meetings and visited him in Damascus during the meeting of the Mediterranean Cardiovascular Society. Due to 9/11, Charlotte and I were unable to again travel to Syria. By then, Sami had become the chief of cardiac surgery at Damascus University. He continued to publish good papers and gave high quality presentations at different meetings. He described and performed the Donald Ross II operation (i.e. replacing the mitral valve with an excised pulmonary artery valve) in good numbers with excellent results.

Sami still is a good friend. He comes to the States to visit his sons, both of whom were educated in this country. Sami told me before the second Iraqi war, "Do not remove Saddam Hussein with force or war, because the balance of power in the Middle East will be disrupted." And so it has been, still now in 2014! His remark turned out to be prophetic.

My year of training at St. Louis University Medical Center went by quickly. I took my oral general surgical boards in the middle of the year and wrote my thoracic boards; I passed both examinations. During the general surgery oral examination, Dr. Arthur Creech gave me a hard time and asked me some very difficult questions about breast surgery; this was during the era of the most radical breast surgeries for breast cancer (mammary chain resections, etc.). Fortunately, the other three oral exam sessions probably compensated for my discussion with Dr. Creech, who was known for heart transplants to the abdominal aortae in rats.

While at St. Louis, I established friendly relations with Drs. Jack Codd, Jim Murphy, and other residents. Nowadays, it is a pleasure to meet them at different professional conferences.

The heart surgeons were influential in cardiology as well and in angiology laboratory and had good relations with Dr. Gerald Mudd, the director of the angiology laboratory. Until that time, left heart catheterization was achieved by left transthoracic puncture of the left atrium, the Brock ventricular puncture, and the so-called Radner puncture. This latter one we used frequently at that time. Free from bleeding disorders or anticoagulation, the patient was laid in the supine position and lightly sedated. A nine-inch #20 gauged needle was entered in the suprasternal area at the sternal notch under local anesthesia and advanced pointing forty-five degrees posteriorly and forty-five degrees left laterally. The first structure entered was the aorta, the second the pulmonary artery and the third the left atrium. Pressures were taken and their shape was thoroughly evaluated. Occasionally the left ventricle was also reached ("shish kabob"). Patients may have been a little sore after this procedure, but we never encountered any major complications and obtained excellent data.

Dr. G. Mudd was an outstanding cardiologist. He may have been the descendant, possibly the grandson, of the Dr. Mudd, who treated Mr. John Wilkes Booth, U.S. President Lincoln's assassin. We never asked Dr. Mudd any questions about his family or possible relations!

In the middle of my year, I was informed by the Committee on Residents Training that I was short in thoracic training and would have to complete another year in thoracic surgery. Of course, this training could not be done at St. Louis University Hospital since it did not have a thoracic training program.

Dr. Hanlon was tremendously helpful with this matter and a few weeks later, suggested two options that I might pursue: I could spend the following year with Dr. Jones, the current president of the American Association for Thoracic Surgery (AATS) in Los Angeles, or I could spend it with Dr. Karl Klassen at Ohio State University in Columbus, Ohio. When I asked Dr. Hanlon which option he would recommend, he chose the one with Dr. Klassen, mentioning that the position was more academic. Thanking Dr. Hanlon, I pursued his recommendation; we moved to Columbus, Ohio. Even today, I am very thankful for Dr. Hanlon's good advice.

My residency training with Dr. Klassen became my most lucrative, beneficial, helpful, and pleasant year of training. We had to move again after just one year in St. Louis, but this seemed to be a minor complication.

St. Louis always was considered as the gateway to the West. The town has a long history, particularly in this regard. It was the place from which Lewis and Clark started their cross-country expedition (1805) on the Missouri-Mississippi, and it was the city in which they finished it upon their return. This city occupied an important southwest key position in U.S.A. in the early 1800s until the Louisiana Purchase was completed in 1805. The first nursing school west of the Mississippi River was established in St. Louis. It also was the city in which Dr. Beaumont practiced (1834) for years after he treated his patient Alexis St. Martin for his chronic gastric fistula. Beaumont contributed a great deal to the physiology of digestion.

At St. Louis University, the Jesuits first appointed civilians rather than priests to the university's board of trustees, whereas at other Catholic universities, only priests served as trustees. Dr. Edward Doisy was working at the university when he received the Nobel Prize for his work on the chemistry of Vitamin K. When I was working at the Fermin Desloge Hospital, Mr. Kurt Schuschnigg, the Austrian Chancellor who resisted Hitler before the annexation of Austria, was lecturing in European history at the university.

In St. Louis, Charlotte and I lived on North Forest Avenue, close to the magnificent Central Park. After a short time, Charlotte started to work in the emergency room of the Barnes-Jewish Hospital. This hospital was within walking distance from our apartment.

One week after arriving in St. Louis, we drove to Jefferson City, the capital city of Missouri, where I took a psychiatric exam required for my medical license, and Charlotte interviewed for her Missouri license. Both of us became very busy in St. Louis with work, but we were happy from then on!

One free weekend, we traveled to the Ozarks in our convertible Mustang. During this trip, we had a close encounter with death when, driving comfortably, we suddenly confronted a huge truck driving towards us in our lane. A young boy without a driver's license was the driver. We had to swerve into the ditch to avoid a collision, but thank God, nothing serious happened to the car or to us, and we survived! In a nice area, we stopped at a Holiday Inn. I walked into the hotel and asked for a room. "We are all full," they answered. Because I knew that this could not true, we stopped at the next public payphone from which I telephoned the same Holiday Inn and introduced myself as Dr. TZL from St. Louis, Missouri. Without any hassles or questions asked, we immediately obtained a reservation at the same Inn, renting a beautiful room for the night.

Lake of the Ozarks has a picturesque and extremely long, curvaceous shoreline. We also visited the neighboring Alton, Illinois, which lies on one of the dammed branches of the Mississippi River. A well-preserved Indian bird is painted on the rocks there.

Culturally, St. Louis was well-developed, with a magnificent orchestra, hockey team, and baseball team. Incidentally, the St. Louis Cardinals had just won the World Series. The construction of the magnificent Gateway to the West or St. Louis Gateway Arch recently had started. It is a huge semicircular structure of significant height (630 feet; 192 meters).

In general, Charlotte and I were happy. We managed to furnish our two-room apartment. I bought a red Dachshund puppy for Charlotte; we named her Tina. She kept us on our toes and chewed the entry door to our apartment. Mr. Israel, the co-owner of the building, warned us that we would have to pay for the door. One day when he was out-of-town, our contracted carpenter repaired the door, and Mr. Israel had to admit that he had been wrong about the door. Afterwards Charlotte and I would laugh about how we had outsmarted Mr. Israel and led him to believe that the door never had been mutilated by our lovely Tina.

At the end of my year, in June 1965, I decided to sit down with Dr. Willman (while Dr. Hanlon was away) and discuss my year's performance. He was relatively reserved, stating that I had done a good job but had a lot to improve. He did not seem to appreciate the differences between the medical systems at Toronto and St. Louis universities. I graciously accepted his criticism, thanked him for all he had done for me, and assured him that I would do my best in Columbus, Ohio.

Ever since, I have found it difficult to understand the mindsets of these physicians towards the training program, their closed and sometime rigid concepts. Analyzing the training of cardiothoracic residents at that time and now, I think I understand the differences.

The training programs should suit the residents, and the teachers should not try to manipulate the whole process to their ultimate convenience and advantage. While the Toronto program was straightforward and made clear what needed to be done, the one in St. Louis was questionable, and what needed to be done was never made clear! The Toronto system was better developed, had a longer history, and aimed for the best development of the trainees. In St. Louis, the "Brownie point" system prevailed, and our work overlapped more with that of the general surgeons. The chief general surgical resident helped with cardiac cases, but the cardiac fellow was not allowed to help with the thoracic cases. The youngest staff members "hung around" to please the seniors, but in the meantime, teaching was delegated to the less senior surgeons.

During the whole year at St. Louis University Medical Center, I do not remember that one visiting professor came to the department, unlike at Toronto and Ohio State Universities. I believe it is an integral responsibility of the training program to acquaint the residents with outstanding surgeons in the same specialty.

Continuous follow-up of residents' progress and development by the Chief (like Professor Kergin in Toronto) definitely was lacking in St. Louis; the half-year discussions about performance were missing. "You were on your own; judge and perform!"

Dr. Willman served as the head of surgery at St. Louis University for twenty-seven years, after Dr. Hanlon left to assume the position of secretary of the American College of Surgeons. In 2009, Dr. Willman had a stroke, developed Alzheimer's in his eighties, and died. Like Dr. E. H. Simmons, who also developed Alzheimer's in his eighties, he was one of my most dynamic teachers. Over ninety years old, Dr. C. R. Hanlon died in May 2011.

Dr. Hanlon given Lifetime Achievement Award

Presiding President LaMar S. McGinnis, Jr., MD, FACS, presented the first Lifetime Achievement Award of the American College of Surgeons (ACS) to C. Rollins Hanlon, MD, FACS, at the Convocation ceremony that preceded the 96th Clinical Congress in Washington, DC.

"It is fitting that the Honors Committee of the College has selected an individual who has devoted a lifetime to his chosen art by not only providing skilled, ethical, and loving care to thousands of surgical patients in his long and illustrious career, but also by serving in many roles and sharing his vast knowledge with our beloved College since becoming a Fellow in 1953." Dr.

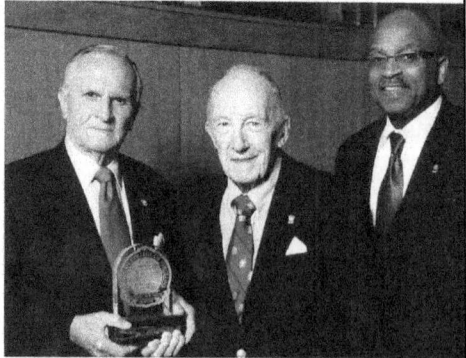

Dr. Hanlon (center) with Dr. McGinnis (left) and L. D. Britt, MD, FACS, current President.

Figure 52. In 2010, Dr. Hanlon received the Lifetime Achievement Award of the American College of Surgeons (ACS).

OHIO STATE UNIVERSITY MEDICAL CENTER: 1965-1966

t the end of June 1965, Charlotte and I packed our belongings into
my leased green Mustang convertible and set out for Columbus,
Ohio. Driving through Indiana, I received a speeding ticket. During my
previous introductory visit, we had leased a nice apartment within
walking distance of the University Hospital.

In order to get a resident's practicing license in Ohio, I had to have an
interview with the Health Commissioner. In 1965, he was ninety-four
years old and by that time, had signed every doctor's practicing license in
Ohio. He gave me a short interview, and the "ceremony" was completed.

Columbus used to be a "cow town;" it is the capital city of Ohio.
Charlotte obtained a job at Columbus's Nationwide Children's Hospital.
Upon our arrival, Dr. Karl Klassen greeted me and showed me to a room,
saying, "This is your office; keep your books and notes here and enjoy it."
My counterpart, Dr. Allen Togut, the first year fellow, arrived later. He
was six feet two inches tall and nervously possessed a steady cough. He

told everybody how it should be in the future. Not a very good surgeon, too slow and mediocre, he never became a hit in chest surgery. Klassen sent us to the July 4th parade; work started the next day. Associates were Drs. Neal Andrews, Charles Meckstrath, and Howard Sirak. Dr. Andrews was the second in command by rank and age. He had the responsibility of taking care of patients in the Ohio State Sanatorium for Tuberculosis (TB), located next door to the Ohio State University Hospital.

Daily operations in the university hospital and operations twice a week in the sanatorium kept us busy. Dr. Andrews was a good surgeon and a gentleman; he was understanding but quite severe; he required good work. After the beginning, he gave me quite a bit of professional freedom. The cases were discussed on a weekly basis with the medical team. Indications for surgery usually warranted a consensus. Dr. Andrews helped with surgery. If the case was tough, he did it himself. Dr. Andrews started to get involved in chemotherapy, when it was not a standard treatment yet. I did over eighty cases of different lung resections, empyemas, and a few thoracoplasties too.

Dr. C. Meckstrath was a solid, good cardiac and thoracic surgeon; he was a kind individual, very interested in teaching. Also a good water skier on the Scioto River, Dr. Sirak was the primary cardiac guy; he was a good surgeon, smart, and imaginative at times. He was trained at Columbia University's Presbyterian Hospital. His problem was that he did not get the cardiac job at this hospital. Dr. James Malm outdid him, having better New York City connections. Chief of Surgery, Dr. Robert Zollinger brought Dr. Sirak to Columbus as the new star, but by now, he had become more interested in collecting paintings. He used to "hop" an airplane to Paris to buy art treasures by Picasso, Monet, or others. Lack of money did not seem to be an obstacle for him; he flew to New Zealand to watch Sir (Dr.) Brian Barratt-Boys do homologous aortic valve replacements. In spite of this remote training, Dr. Sirak never did one of these operations during my training in Columbus.

Operating at the Ohio State Sanatorium for Tuberculosis was not a problem for us. As a sanitary and preventative measure, we showered after visiting this institution! However, if we encountered a case of unexpected tuberculosis in the main hospital, it always created havoc. During that year, I completed over eighty major cases there. The next year tuberculosis was disappearing, and they had only fifteen to twenty operations. Afterwards, the Ohio State Sanatorium for Tuberculosis was closed permanently.

One of the most decorated surgeons of the American College of Surgeons and president of all prestigious societies, Dr. Robert Zollinger described "Zollinger-Ellison" syndrome. At that time, treatment of the proven syndrome was unequivocally total gastrectomy. Zollinger already suspected that it may be a part of a multiple endocrine syndrome.

Dr. Zollinger was a "benign" terror! Usually he fired one or two residents a year; he sent them home for several days to be scared and think about their futures. Zollinger usually called them back to work after four or five days. When he was out of town, every evening he would telephone the resident on call, requiring a complete rundown on the patients; he then would give his orders (i.e. what to do in the next twenty-four hours). Grand rounds were a great show every Saturday. Everybody had to be there on time. The format often changed, and the criticism was cruel.

One Saturday morning I was doing a bronchoscopy when Dr. Zollinger came through the operating room. He proceeded to chew me out for operating during grand rounds. One Sunday morning, I was finishing my chart dictations, when Dr. Z. appeared and asked why the charts were not dictated. I told him I just finished them. "No. Why are the charts of your attendings not done?" he asked me. I told him that it was not my responsibility. "Not your charts, but your attendings' charts," he said. "You are responsible for ensuring that your attending physicians do their charts on time." To avoid unnecessary reprimands, I tried to encourage my attending physicians to do their charts on time.

Early mornings started with rounds; we were in the operating room by quarter to eight. If we were twenty minutes late, Klassen already was "in the chest" of the first case; he often did two or three cases in the morning, but most certainly was on the golf course in the afternoon. Every chest case was a beautiful teaching case. Closed heart cases often were a problem, though. A technique did not exist to obtain chamber pressures on the left side of the heart. The cardiologists were conducting a study to record sounds—echoes—with direct probes in the heart chamber. This procedure was cumbersome and at times it created bleeding spots.

I called Dr. Klassen's attention to the fact that I had done several Radner's Punctures (Percutaneous Suprasternal Punctures). He supervised me doing one of these procedures in the operating room, and then he told me to "go-ahead" for selected cases. This continued for about twenty procedures without any complications, until the cardiologists (specifically Dr. Wooley) raised objections to this "brutal" technique. That was the end of Radner's punctures; we also did not collect direct pressures. The cases were very good with excellent results, and I was getting along very well. Dr. Klassen was wonderful. If I made a mistake, he used to say, "I should have told you to watch for that particular problem."

It was difficult to get blood to fully prime the pump (i. e. heart-lung machine). In order to resolve this problem, Dr. Sirak used to consecutively book two patients with the same blood type. The pump was kept full after the first, case and the same blood was used for the second case. Of course, shortly thereafter, Dr. Cooley developed hemodilution, which instantly significantly reduced the blood requirements. At that time, we knew nothing about HIV; every patient was tested for syphilis. This technique was not appealing and proved to be "unhygienic!"

One day after a crash, a motorcyclist was brought to the Emergency Room in moribund condition. Staff was not able to intubate him. We were called; I performed a tracheostomy. The patient's trachea was completely transected. I had to put my finger in the distal part of the trachea to find it, and we subsequently intubated the patient's distal trachea. When he was stabilized in a few days, I performed a tracheal end-to-end anastomosis with Dr. Manuel Tzagournis. After the motorcyclist's full recovery, both of the patient's vocal cords were paralyzed, and Dr. Tzagournis had to pin both arytenoids. The patient fully recovered and was discharged home.

One day, I explored a patient for possible left pneumonectomy. He was unresectable, but we had to have a tissue diagnosis. Dr. Klassen always insisted on tissue biopsies; he used to say, "The patient was sent to us for us to make a diagnosis; we have to make one based on tissue biopsies." I made a cautious tissue excision and sent it to pathology. The "pathologist" called and stated: "This biopsy was not enough to make a diagnosis of no cancer." I made a more generous biopsy and sent this one to pathology. The same statement came from the pathologist. The third biopsy caused major bleeding in the patient, and I had to deal with it over three hours. The pathologist called with a diagnosis, "Carcinoma." The Chief, Dr. O. had a look at all three specimens, and each one was diagnosed as cancerous! "Thank you." Fortunately after several hours of stitching and holding the area (i.e. the pulmonary artery), the patient survived the biopsies.

Hormone-producing, small cell, "oat cell" carcinoma already was known in the literature. We did a right upper lobectomy for one carcinoma that was less than two centimeters. The patient died a few weeks later, likely due to hypokalemia and cardiac complications.

One of Dr. Klassen's patients was diagnosed with carcinoma of the esophagus, which was one centimeter and incidentally found. He underwent a smooth esophagogastrectomy. While recovering on the sixth day, during a bowel movement, he collapsed and died of massive pulmonary embolism.

Dr. Klassen had a long-standing dispute with Dr. Groves of the Cleveland Clinic about esophageal perforation; he insisted that certain forms of perforation can be treated conservatively, without an operation, with good results. Dr. Groves never acknowledged this possibility, to treat perforations without operations. The debate between the two men was continuous. As of 2011, more and more articles in the literature suggest treating perforations without operations. Dr. Klassen had been right. I became very familiar with conservative treatment, and I became an expert, utilizing this experience in my later practice. Dr. H. Soutar and others designed plastic tubes that were tried without much success in cases of unresectable carcinoma of the esophagus.

We had several visiting professors on the service. Dr. Klassen's teaching philosophy proved to be exceptional. He always said, "Dr. So-and-So is coming. He will spend a half-day with you. You are responsible!" Take Dr. Steel, for instance. We residents showed cases to him, asking for his views on treatments. We "picked his brain." We, the residents, met and engaged with a great number of "famous" thoracic surgeons. Later while practicing and teaching in Buffalo, New York, I implemented Klassen's teaching philosophy.

At this point in my narrative, I would like to digress somewhat and relate a few sad stories.

Dr. J.P.M. III was one of the senior general surgical residents; he was a very bright and smart fellow. He experimented on dogs, trying to coagulate their induced lung tumors by laser ablation. By doing so, he expected to do some immunological studies too, titrating and watching the tumors' recurrence. One year after I left Ohio State, I heard that Dr. J.P.M. III died after being involved in a bad car accident. What a loss! Today, radiofrequency coagulation is applied in some stage-one lung tumor cases for the same reason, to induce immunological resistance.

Dr. M. was a young, upcoming, "progressive," attending vascular surgeon. He and his wife always flew on separate airplanes; they explained their rationale for traveling separately in terms of an airplane crash—if such a tragedy were to occur and one of them perished in such an accident, the other spouse would survive and be able to raise their children. Dr. M. developed acute leukemia and died shortly before the age of forty.

Dr. Carl Klassen was without a doubt my best teacher and chief. Considerate and most supportive of the residents, he would stand up for his residents any time. He took good care of us.

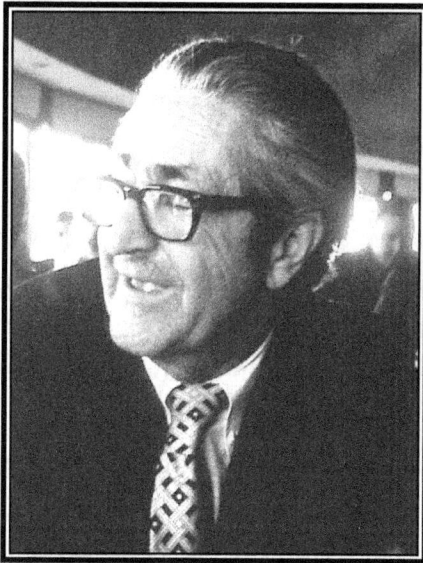

Figure 53. Dr. Karl Klassen

Spring 1966 was in full swing. I still did not have a permanent job, and my fellowship board exam was approaching quickly. I saw a journal advertisement for a three-month locum as a National Parks doctor at Glacier National Park in Montana. I wrote a letter of inquiry, but I did not get an answer. In early June, in a state of "desperation," I telephoned the doctor in Whitefish, Montana, who was responsible for supplying medical coverage for the park. Apologetic, she mentioned that they never received my letter. The spring floods had washed away the railway tracks, and my letter probably had been lost in the Flathead River. She said that they already had employed an elderly doctor for the job.

No job!

I tried not to panic.

In the middle of June, during the third week, this time I received a desperate telephone call from this doctor, "Could you start work here in July?" she asked, "The elderly doctor has sustained a myocardial infarction, and we are without anybody to provide medical coverage in the park." What great luck! I would be able to spend the summer in the Rockies doing an easy job, while studying for my boards and taking care of my pregnant wife Charlotte. My guardian angel had rescued me again!

In the training process that we residents underwent at that time, it was always necessary to be available at all times, to work hard, and to be pleasant. If a serendipitous opportunity presented itself, you had to grab it! This was the nature of the "game" of medicine at that time. Carpe Viam (Seize the Road)! It was not enough to have luck; it was just as important to take the opportunity, if it was given!

Shortly after I left Ohio State, one or two years later, I heard that Dr. Klassen was diagnosed with pancreatic carcinoma. Dr. Zollinger had explored him but could not do anything. Carl asked for one dose of 6000 rads (R) radiation, which he received, but he died within months of the diagnosis. He will be remembered by his residents for a long time!

GLACIER NATIONAL PARK, MONTANA: THE "WILD WEST"

After I was offered the park doctor job at Glacier National Park on very short notice, Charlotte and I abruptly departed from Columbus. We bid a thankful farewell to my chiefs, and at the end of June, we packed up our less than one-year-old green Ford Mustang and headed west with our one-and-a-half-year-old red, short-haired Dachshund Tina. We never returned to Columbus, even though we had very friendly relationships with the people there with whom we were connected and worked. C'est la vie (That's life).

While in St. Louis, I had started to have expensive problems with my Austin Healey Sprite, and heeding my father-in-law's advice, we leased a brand new Mustang for two years. The Mustang was one of the first cars produced by Ford as a new design. I should have kept it. Now it would be a very valuable and precious antique car. Because I never seemed to have an extra penny to spend and always seemed to be on the move, eventually we got rid of the Mustang too!

The weather in the Midwest that summer was brilliant but extremely hot. While driving, we had to use our air-conditioning almost all the time, and Tina had to be wrapped in a cold, water-soaked towel. On the way, we visited the Badlands National Park (this terrain looks like the moon surface with canyons) and Mount Rushmore National Memorial in South Dakota, where we viewed the sculpted heads of the four presidents. In two days we had made it to the capital of Montana, Helena, where I visited the state health department. I had to report there to get my temporary state medical license. From here, we traveled to Yellowstone National Park, where we camped in our pup tent. The nights were so cold that in the mornings, a thin rim of ice lined the shore of the campground's rivulet. The Yellowstone National Park was splendid: the Old Faithful geyser never failed to entertain us; the wildlife roamed the roads, and bears scavenged among tourists for food.

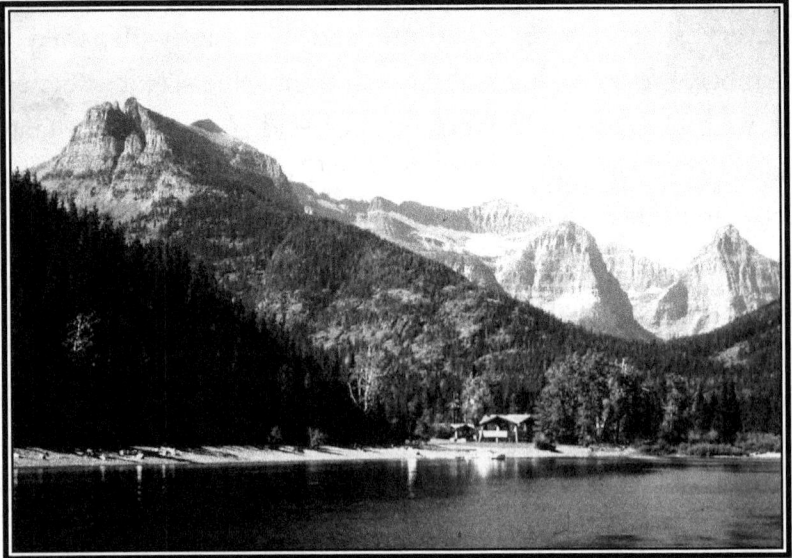

Figure 54. A photograph of Glacier National Park that I took in July or August 1966.

222

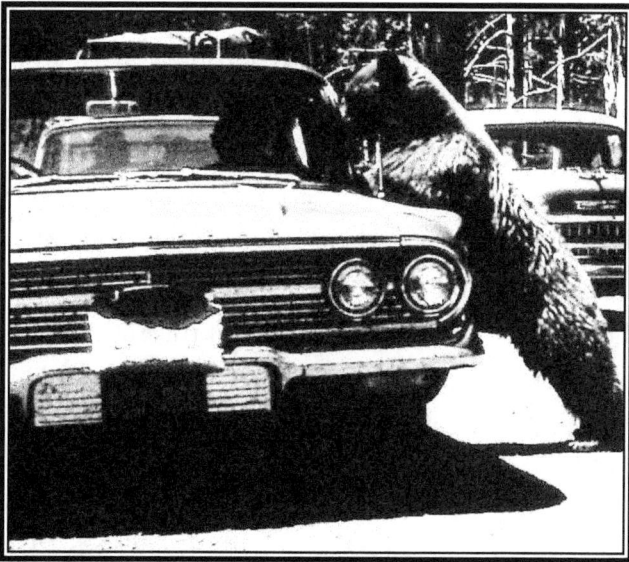

Figure 55. Yellowstone National Park in the summer of 1966: bears and wild animals roamed freely in the park. In this photograph, a bear stands against a car window looking for some food.

Some of the visitors fed food scraps to these huge beasts. This behavior was truly stupid. Considering the bear attacks during the summers, it was foolish for tourists to try to feed these animals. Today these types of dangerous thrills are discouraged in the national parks.

After driving another 400 miles, we arrived in Whitefish, Montana, where I reported to Dr. McIntosh, the official responsible for coordinating medical services in Glacier National Park. My duties involved providing alternating medical coverage in the Lake McDonald area for three days and then in the East Glacier Park Lodge area for another three days. We received a room and food each time we checked in for a three-day stay.

The drive from one area of coverage to the other, about eighty to one hundred miles from one lodge to the other, could be completed in one of two ways:

- By driving south along the notorious Flathead River, where mountain goats could be seen at the salt lick, and then curving north to East Glacier.
- By driving through the spectacular "Highway to the Sun," the serpentine Logan Pass, to the east side; it was a two-lane highway. The outer lane was near to the edge of the road, which dropped hundreds or thousands of feet below. When cars have driven off this pass, they were left in the steep gullies of this rugged mountain pass, probably because they could not be retrieved from below. The views along this pass were spectacular, but one had to be careful not to be mesmerized by them while driving.

Moose could be spotted early in the morning in Lake McDonald valley and grizzly bears midway up on the pass. After a rotation between the two areas, I had one free day from work during which I could go hiking or driving to the neighboring towns.

The hotel offices were well-equipped for handling outpatient services, including the medical care of cuts, blisters, ticks, sunburns, and other minor injuries. I spent the eight hours when I was on-call in the office, but when I was not on eight-hour shift duty, I had to be readily available any time including at night for emergencies. The time I spent in the office gave me an excellent chance to study for my thoracic boards. During these hours, my wife Charlotte walked, socialized, read, chatted with the nurse, if the nurse was free, and enjoyed the fresh, unpolluted air. Charlotte was six-months pregnant with our first child. We usually managed to lunch together in the lodge dining room.

I was searching for a permanent cardiothoracic job during these months. Some offers looked good, and some, less attractive. I thought I had a good chance to get a position in Edmonton, Canada, with Dr. John Callaghan, but the opportunity dissipated, when I was not notified that he gave the job to another person. When I inquired about the status of my job application, Callaghan did not have the courtesy to update me himself; rather his secretary told me that I had not been chosen. Feeling slighted, I had expected a "swollen-headed," conceited, cardiac chief surgeon to behave in a more gentlemanlike and fair way toward me. How wrong I was!

Somehow I heard that Queen's University in Kingston, Ontario, was looking for a cardiothoracic surgeon. I contacted them, and eventually, I was invited to interview for the job. In early August, Charlotte shuttled me to Great Falls (Montana) Airport for my interview trip. In order to get to Great Falls, we had to drive through an Indian reservation notorious for excessive drinking. According to federal law, when a new couple gets married in this reservation, the newlyweds receive a bull and several cows from the government to start their productive lives. Of course, at the wedding, there is always a great pow-wow and often the participants slaughter several new cows to feed the wedding guests. During this month when Charlotte and I drove through the village, they slaughtered the single bull they received—no further breeding of the animals was possible.

When I interviewed at Queen's University in Kingston, my reception was rather welcoming. By now my friend Dr. Ernie Sterns was on staff in general surgery at the University Hospital. The cardiothoracic department had one surgeon, Dr. R. Beverly Lynn. He had completed some training with Dr. Melrose at the Royal Postgraduate Medical School, in London, United Kingdom. Dr. Lynn was very friendly; he informed me that he planned to retire in the near future. I also visited Hotel Dieu Hospital, the other hospital in Kingston. They promised to put me on staff there too, if I was offered the Queen's University position. If I recall correctly, I also had an interview with the new dean of the School of Medicine at Queen's University, Dr. E. Harry Botterell, the previous chief of neurosurgery of the University of Toronto.

In his previous position, he had been very well-respected as a surgeon and chief but was dreaded for his stern and unapproachable attitude. Dr. Botterell behaved just the opposite with me, and when I left Kingston, I had the feeling that I would get the job. A few weeks later, I was offered the job, and I was informed that I needed to start to work sometime in the middle of September. This was marvelous news, since it meant that I would not be unemployed after training for so many years! The first job post-training is almost never the last one, but it usually gives the new medical professional the chance to "get in the groove" and start his or her career. My surgical career had been launched!

Meanwhile, the days flew by for me at Glacier National Park. My work there was easy, and I used the time to study for my boards. On my free days, I went hiking, traveling, photographing, and sightseeing. The beauty of the park was unbelievable to me; the park reminded me of the European Alps more than any of the other national parks in the Rockies. The wildlife was abundant; the terrain was a photographer's dream. When I was off duty, I took long hikes, sometimes twenty-five to thirty miles on trails through passes and descents.

One morning at East Glacier, we heard a gunshot and then saw an Indian pelting the brown bear he just had shot. Indians arre allowed to hunt anywhere.

We drove north to Kintla Lakes, hoping to see grizzly bears, but we only spotted some huge footprints. Driving on a dirt road uphill, a fully-loaded lorry proceeded ahead of us. Suddenly the driver must have lost control, and the lorry started to roll backwards toward us. In order to avoid a major crash, I had to put my Mustang in reverse and drive backwards at full speed on the narrow road. After several hundred yards, the truck stopped, and we avoided another major accident. A very close call, the second one involving this car!

One day, we drove to Banff, Alberta, Canada, passing by the beautiful Waterton Lakes National Park and the Prince of Wales Hotel (the Canadian part of Glacier National Park). Further north, Banff was spectacular: the lodge at Lake Louise sits on the shore like a majestic castle. Opposite it, the glacier drains and makes the lake. On the other side of the town, cable cars shuttle visitors to the mountaintop, from which during the summer, they can see seventeen active glaciers.

One day while we were having a drink at the bar, we chatted with the CEO of East Glacier. He inquired about our satisfaction with the accommodations, food, and services. We confirmed that we were delighted with them; we described the experience as "just like that of a honeymoon." Concluding that we just had gotten married, the CEO looked at Charlotte's enlarged waistline, smiled, and commented, "Don't worry. I was in the same situation when I got married." We laughed, but Charlotte did not appreciate his response.

With "broken hearts," we left Glacier National Park, where we had had so much fun and spent two beautiful months. Luckily, Charlotte's pregnancy had proceeded without complications. We agreed that we wanted to return to this beautiful place, and we did more than thirty years later, after 2000.

On Labor Day weekend 1966, we started to drive back to Toronto in the Mustang; it took two-and-a-half days of hard driving to get there. We then drove to Kingston to rent an apartment on the top floor of a fancy apartment tower next to the yacht club on the shore of Kingston Harbor.

EPILOGUE:
PAST, PRESENT, AND FUTURE

⌘

Over time, I often thought of my journey to freedom. The more I analyzed it, the more it became incredible. How did I manage to achieve academic excellence and success in my profession without any outside help? Gradually, I became inspired to write about my journey.

My life in the totalitarian system did not allow for any compromises, and especially in the communist era, it became unbearable. This time mostly included my university years. I had to face the realities in Hungary and determine my future. I was truly lucky that the once-in-a-lifetime, three-month "window" of opportunity presented itself to me, that I "seized" this "opportunity" (Carpe Diem), and that I was able to escape from Hungary in 1956.

The very moment I crossed the Iron Curtain, I knew that unlimited opportunities would present themselves; however, failure and downfall were as possible as success in my future. Like Odysseus in the great epic poem of the *Odyssey*, I had to navigate "between Charybdis and Scylla," but with hard work and most of the time with the right choices, I managed to settle down into a successful medical practice, in Buffalo, NY, USA, during the age of pioneering discoveries in heart surgery.

By that time, my lovely wife Charlotte and I also were establishing our family. Luckily, we had three healthy children, a boy followed by two beautiful girls. With Charlotte always with me and supporting me, we had an unforgettable, happy 49 years together. We shared life together and came through the "bumps" together, eventually victoriously. To remember those years and rekindle them is my greatest joy nowadays.

My grown children are my ultimate happiness, and I have the chance to talk to them every day, sometimes several times a day; they always curiously ask me, "Dad, what is new?"

Paul is doing "cutting-edge" vascular surgery, and he skis with me when he has time.

Cheryl is an indispensable help with my writing and particularly with this book. She read its various drafts and versions and helped me to edit it. Without her assistance, this book would not be here. She wishes that she could obtain a job closer.

Laura continues to juggle full-time and part-time employment opportunities as well as her various professional responsibilities.

I have to somewhat digress here and mention the economy and Obamacare, because I believe they are very significant to the future of this country, its young people, and the practice of medicine. With Obamacare gradually being phased in, and its consequences remaining unresolved, companies do not like to offer full-time employment with health benefits to employees. This is a very unfortunate development that has many sad and disastrous repercussions for families and ultimately for this country. The future of medicine under Obamacare remains unknown, unless major revisions will take place.

To write the story of my "desertion" from Hungary has been on my mind for a long time. The choice of my specialty, cardiovascular surgery, and its exploding development focused all my attention to the changes right from the beginning.

While the early sixties were the time of pioneering discoveries and surgical techniques, the seventies represented the stabilization and development of standard techniques, with major improvements and refinements. Slowly, minimally invasive procedures took over the field of cardiovascular surgery. Operating on the beating heart, surgeons use retrograde catheter techniques as today's standard treatments. Research focusing on the outcomes and financial reimbursements gratifies the cautious surgeons, who have better results than their predecessors. Nationalized medicine crept in; the "knight" surgeons became "knaves," and they have to watch so as to avoid becoming "pawns." These are really revolutionary times in medicine, and we have to preserve, by all means, primarily the patients' rights.

The changes came so fast that they outgrew the well-trained surgeons in no time. Postgraduate education— standardized for many years—had to be modified too.

As they do in other medical specialties, many changes in cardiac and thoracic surgery continue to occur. New techniques require "hands-on sessions" and simulation courses of retrograde techniques, etc. Electrophysiology is not in the surgeon's hands anymore. Cardiovascular critical care is becoming a new specialty. Postgraduate education broke away from the "classical" teachings of mentors.

Modern medicine has to be reconsidered based on the Hippocratic principle: "primum non nocere" (First, do no harm).

At the end of my full professional practice, in the final analysis, I still may say that if I would start again, I still would do cardiac surgery. It has been an incredible journey.

PART V
APPENDICES

APPENDIX 1
PROFESSOR CHARLES GATI'S BOOK ON THE HUNGARIAN REVOLUTION OF 1956: PRECONCEIVED IDEAS

~⟐~

On the fiftieth anniversary of the Hungarian Revolution, in 2006, a Hungarian by the name of Mr. Charles Gati, a professor at Johns Hopkins University, published a book titled *Failed Illusions: Moscow, Washington, Budapest, and the 1956 Hungarian Revolt*, in which he analyzed the events of the revolution and concluded that the revolution could have been averted by negotiations. *Johns Hopkins Magazine* then published an essay on Gati's book. In response to this essay, I wrote to the Editor of the *Johns Hopkins Magazine*.

Below I include my letter to the Editor of the *Johns Hopkins Magazine*, and my comments follow.

MY LETTER TO THE EDITOR
OF THE *JOHNS HOPKINS MAGAZINE*
"THE OTHER PRECONCEIVED IDEAS VERSUS THE TRUTH"
BY T. Z. LAJOS, M.D.

The *John Hopkins Magazine* regularly has been sent to me, maybe because one of my children graduated from The Johns Hopkins University. The September 2006 issue published an article on page 30, under Wholly Hopkins, subtitled: "History: The Hungarian Revolt Reconsidered."

This article was written by Professor Charles Gati, who is distinguished by his previous studies and who is at present a Senior Adjunct Professor at the Nietze School of Advanced International Studies at Hopkins.

I must say that I read the article with disappointment. This article was based on his studies and supported by his book entitled *Failed Illusions: Moscow, Washington, Budapest, and the 1956 Hungarian Revolt.* Gati clearly declared his stance on the Hungarian Revolution in 2006; he stated that there was a chance for negotiation in 1956. All I can say is that any political issue always has a chance for reconsideration fifty years later. In later times, reconsiderations usually result in disagreements, delays, arguments, different opinions, no decisions, and no support. One cannot do anything about it anyway!

These ideas of Mr. Gati seem to be proven wrong right from the beginning! The country and the university students wanted primarily and unconditionally: "Ruskies, [Russians] go home!" At 3 p.m. on Monday, October 22, 1956, the students of the Budapest Technical University published a "Manifesto" of sixteen points, before the start of the uprising. (See Appendix 3, which includes a complete copy of the Demonstrators' Manifesto) Point 1. of the Manifesto stated: "We demand the immediate evacuation of all Soviet troops, in conformity with the provisions of the Treaty of Peace."

This first point of the Manifesto became universally the first and most important slogan of the Revolution: "Ruskies, go home!"

Mr. Gati made a point: "the Soviet Union was not eager for a military solution." This personal opinion is highly debatable based on the existing contract among the "Warsaw Pact" nations and the philosophy, doctrine, and policy of the Soviet Union. He suggested that the USSR "did not like what was happening, and it wanted to regain its authority, but it was prepared to negotiate." This was not true; negotiating was nothing but a "delaying tactic" and a "trap," which was followed by the liquidation and arrests of key figures, including the Hungarian Prime Minister Mr. Imre Nagy.

I have no idea where Mr. Gati obtained these misconceptions. The communists used these policies to obtain time, to resolve their own squabbles, to devise their strategies, and to organize their troops. The phone calls and initially the rather "hot" discussions between Mr. Gero, who previously specialized in terrorist activities in Spain, Yuri Andropov, the Soviet Ambassador to Hungary, Marshal Georgy Zhukov, the hero of the Soviet Union, and Nikita Khrushchev clearly showed some delay of decisions but definitely not wavering. Anastas Mikoyan, the Machiavellian Armenian, was the only person in the Kremlin hierarchy who wanted to negotiate throughout the whole crisis. He and Mikhail Suslov were sent to Budapest to assess the situation after the initial success of the revolution (Oct. 24-Nov. 4, 1956). On their return, when the decision for Soviet military attack already had been made, he (Mikoyan) was frustrated and unsuccessfully argued with Khrushchev; Mikoyan was against military intervention in Hungary.

The political scene did not change for another forty years after the Soviets cruelly crushed the Hungarian Revolution, until President Ronald Reagan told Gorbachev to "tear down" the Berlin wall. By this time the Soviet Union already was disintegrating. The Soviet Union never negotiated seriously while the Berlin wall existed; the Iron Curtain stood firmly, and the Warsaw Pact's agreement was followed by its nations, since it was sealed early in 1956.

Lenin said, "Only equals may come to an agreement." But for the Soviets, Hungarians were not equal!

Professor Gati severely criticized Imre Nagy for initially failing to recognize the legitimacy of the national revolution and for later, when he was prime minister, embracing the most radical goals of the revolution. Of course, Professor Gati seemed to ignore the fact that Imre Nagy was appointed as the prime minister almost right before the events, and he was the one who wanted to negotiate and to prevent bloodshed. The request for withdrawal of Soviet troops was made after his appointment.

As far as international situations are concerned, I agree that the CIA lacked preparation, and U.S. policymakers were not interested in getting involved with the Hungarian events. The Eisenhower administration's "roll back policy prevailed." I do not agree with Gati and his absurd claim that "the primary interest was to divert the funds through Asia because of the Korean War." President Eisenhower and his Secretary of State, John Foster Dulles, revealed the United States' primary interest when they focused on the Suez Canal situation.

Professor Gati seemed to ignore the fact that the free shipping of the modern world was endangered at that point by the Suez Canal crisis, created by Gamel Nasser nationalizing the canal and taking full control of shipping. Sir Anthony Eden had to resign, due to his own aggressive attitude as British prime minister. The American neutrality was obvious even in this "second" world crisis. Finally, the United Nations involved the Canadian Prime Minister Lester Pearson as a chief negotiator. (He received the Nobel Peace Prize for his efforts). War was averted with his diplomatic skills and efforts. For weeks, the United Nations' Security Council did not even bring up the discussion of the Hungarian Revolution and Russia's military intervention in a foreign country. The decision of the National Assembly of the United Nations was powerless and impotent when it was made in later months. There is no question that the Suez Canal crisis dominated the attention of the press, because of its high stakes--the future political, economic, and commercial interests of the free world. It was a major factor turning the attention of the free world away from the Hungarian Revolution.

Andropov, Mikoyan, and Suslov were the ones to assess the situation, and the Soviets had absolutely no intention of negotiating. Why does Mr. Gati think that a satellite nation such as Hungary, which was a member of the Warsaw Pact nations, would have been freed from the communist political sphere and the Warsaw Pact Nations?

The plan to crush the revolution by the Soviets shrewdly was discussed in the Kremlin. The decision was made in spite of the objection of Mr. Mikoyan, who had just returned from Budapest, and it irritated Mr. Khrushchev before his special, hurried journey with his commissaries to the Warsaw Pact countries and to Tito's Yugoslavia, to explain the rationale for military interventions.

Prior to this trip, China's Chairman Mao Tsetung also was consulted at least twice. The Chairman had a definite opinion on the Hungarian Revolution, which was well documented later in his "Red Book." (See the paragraph on the "Correct handling of contradictions among the people," February 27, 1957, First Pocket edition, page 57). The Chairman clearly expressed the communist ideology of the Communist nations and its dictatorships regarding the Hungarian Revolt as follows:

It (the revolutionary rebellion in Hungary in 1956) was a case of reactionaries inside the socialist country in league with imperialists, attempting to achieve the conspiratorial aims by taking advantage of contradictions among the people to form dissension and stir-up disorder. This lesson of the Hungarian events merits attention.

(Mao Tsetung, page 57)

These events and statements do not go along with Gati's opinion: the "Soviet Union was not eager for a military solution."

The mighty Soviet Union also suppressed "minor" revolutionary efforts in the satellite nations before, such as in Czechoslovakia (the Dubcek Revolution) and in Poland (Poznan; the Polish workers at Gdansk). These peaceful demonstrations did not gain any victory until the Soviet Union itself almost fully fell apart.

In the political world there is always another way; there always will be criticisms of events, suggestions for us that we should learn. Explosive revolutions like the Hungarian Revolution of 1956 did not work that way. Well proven by the defeat of previous Hungarian uprisings like Kossuth's in 1848, even Count István Széchenyi and his party's "ready to negotiate policy" and peace initiatives did not change the revolutionary events in 1848.

Finally, it is shameful and distasteful to express conciliatory philosophy and opinion during the fifty-year anniversary of the Hungarian Revolution, considering the heroic fights and lost lives of the Hungarian freedom fighters for freedom and democracy. President George W. Bush visited the country in 2006 to make a point of this historic, heroic event.

Professor Gati's previous employment is highly suggestive that he obtained these preconceived ideas some time previously, while working as a reporter in training for the *Magyar Nemzet, a* communist newspaper by this time, totally under communist censure.

But finally, I also should add, that I totally disagree with Gati's statement: "Americans and Hungarians alike should be ready to take a moralistic and therefore a more self-critical look at what they did, how their mistakes contributed to the revolution's downfall, and what else they could have done." What were the "mistakes?" Would it have helped if Americans and Hungarians took this moralistic, self-critical look?

MY COMMENTS

My response to the Editor of the *John Hopkins Magazine* is documented above. The general comments and criticisms regarding Gati's book justifiably were very negative, and it was felt that Mr. Gati's "work" was filled with "preconceived ideas."

How can an intelligent person like Gati enumerate on the events of the Revolution and claim that negotiations would have worked? Totally absurd!

My letter to the Editor was ignored; it never was published. I was not even thanked for my time or interest! Obviously, the politics of "higher" authorities prevailed.

APPENDIX 2
THE FOUR PILLARS OF
REVOLUTION

In my estimation, four crucial, fundamental "pillars" of revolution were present in Hungary in 1956 and provided the foundations for the Hungarian Revolution:

• Political- a totalitarian dictatorship existed in Hungary!
• Religious- the materialistic, atheistic beliefs of the regime as well as its Bolshevik ideology served as the regime's bases for preserving the status quo under communism in Hungary;
• Desire for change- segments of the population strongly desired economic change and wanted to eliminate the consequences of years of exploitation.
• Desire to eradicate foreign occupation and oppression- the definite, immediate goal was to rid Hungary of its foreign occupiers: "Ruskies, [Russians] go home," the demonstrators chanted.

The Hungarian uprising brewed for several years; the question was not if it would occur, but rather when would the time come?

APPENDIX 3
THE DEMONSTRATORS'
MANIFESTO:
OCTOBER 22, 1956

Two days before the Revolution began in Hungary, the demonstrators drafted the following Manifesto:

1. We demand the immediate evacuation of all Soviet troops, in conformity with the provisions of the Peace Treaty.

2. We demand the election by secret ballot of all Party members from top to bottom, and of new officers for the lower, middle and upper echelons of the Hungarian Workers Party. These officers shall convene a Party Congress as early as possible in order to elect a Central Committee.

3. A new Government must be constituted under the direction of Imre Nagy: all criminal leaders of the Stalin-Rákosi era must be immediately dismissed.

4. We demand public enquiry into the criminal activities of Mihály Farkas and his accomplices. Mátyás Rákosi, who is the person most responsible for crimes of the recent past as well as for our country's ruin, must be returned to Hungary for trial before a people's tribunal.

5. We demand general elections by universal, secret ballot are held throughout the country to elect a new National Assembly, with all political parties participating. We demand that the right of workers to strike be recognised.

6. We demand revision and re-adjustment of Hungarian-Soviet and

Hungarian-Yugoslav relations in the fields of politics, economics and cultural affairs, on a basis of complete political and economic equality, and of non-interference in the internal affairs of one by the other.

7. We demand the complete reorganisation of Hungary's economic life under the direction of specialists. The entire economic system, based on a system of planning, must be re-examined in the light of conditions in Hungary and in the vital interest of the Hungarian people.

8. Our foreign trade agreements and the exact total of reparations that can never be paid must be made public. We demand to be precisely informed of the uranium deposits in our country, on their exploitation and on the concessions to the Russians in this area. We demand that Hungary have the right to sell her uranium freely at world market prices to obtain hard currency.

9. We demand complete revision of the norms operating in industry and an immediate and radical adjustment of salaries in accordance with the just requirements of workers and intellectuals. We demand a minimum living wage for workers.

10. We demand that the system of distribution be organised on a new basis and that agricultural products be utilised in rational manner. We demand equality of treatment for individual farms.

11. We demand reviews by independent tribunals of all political and economic trials as well as the release and rehabilitation of the innocent. We demand the immediate repatriation of prisoners of war (World War II) and of civilian deportees to the Soviet Union, including prisoners sentenced outside Hungary.

12. We demand complete recognition of freedom of opinion and of expression, of freedom of the press and of radio, as well as the creation of a daily newspaper for the MEFESZ Organisation (Hungarian

Federation of University and College Students' Associations).

13. We demand that the statue of Stalin, symbol of Stalinist tyranny and political oppression, be removed as quickly as possible and be replaced by a monument in memory of the martyred freedom fighters of 1848-49.

14. We demand the replacement of emblems foreign to the Hungarian people by the old Hungarian arms of Kossuth. We demand new uniforms for the Army which conform to our national traditions. We demand that March 15 be declared a national holiday and that the October 6th be a day of national mourning on which schools will be closed.

15. The students of the Technological University of Budapest declare unanimously their solidarity with the workers and students of Warsaw and Poland in their movement towards national independence.

16. The students of the Technological University of Budapest will organise as rapidly as possible local branches of MEFESZ, and they have decided to convene at Budapest, on Saturday October 27, a Youth Parliament at which all the nation's youth shall be represented by their delegates.

APPENDIX 4
THE KOSSUTH REVOLUTION IN HUNGARY:
1848

In general, people, including historians, often compare the two Hungarian revolutions to each other: the 1848 revolution led by Lajos Kossuth and the 1956 people's uprising. These comparisons are misguided because they attempt to compare two totally different events to each other.

Kossuth 's uprising was against the Habsburg regime, which failed to meet the nationalistic objectives of Hungary. While the 1956 revolution had all the pillars of a revolution, the 1848 uprising was missing some of the four principal elements:

• The Habsburg era was *not* based upon a dictatorial, totalitarian regime.
• Religious elements never played a role.
• Economics played a minor part.
• While Hungary may have lacked total independence, the Habsburgs were not foreign occupiers.

While both revolutions were defeated with the help of the Russians, this fact does not in itself justify comparing the two events. This is not the place to give a detailed analysis and comparison of the two uprisings!

APPENDIX 5
FESTSCHRIFT IN HONOR OF DR.
EDWARD H. SIMMONS

On May 9, 2009, Dr. Edward H. Simmons passed away after a protracted illness. I was deeply saddened by the news of Ed's death. He had been my lifelong mentor and friend for more than fifty years.

My lifelong relationship with Ed Simmons began in 1958, when I had the privilege to assist him with one of his first menesectomies. I had difficulty understanding the fast-talking but unquestionably brilliant, young, Canadian, orthopedic surgeon, who had just returned from his travels, facilitated by the McLaughlin Traveling Fellowship. Because I had arrived to Canada from a foreign country a few months earlier, my language skills were "raw," and I was unfamiliar with the vocabularies and terminologies of the North American medicine and postgraduate training programs.

I became known as "Tom zee Bum" and was given the opportunity to work on Ed's orthopedic surgery service for six months, since his other attending surgeons did not care for my assistance as a foreign, junior resident. Ed's fast moving clinical service and his challenging approaches stimulated my dedication, loyalty, and unrivaled support for this brilliant man.

At that time, the challenges of back surgery, especially surgical correction of ankylosing spondylitis, seemed to be insurmountable, but not for Ed Simmons, who successfully pioneered intraoperative and postoperative approaches to the complications faced by these patients. These patients often had tracheostomies prior to orthopedic surgery and postoperatively remained on Stryker frames for weeks.

The excruciating pain of arthritic knee was another type of case requiring a "cutting-edge," surgical approach. Ed pioneered the solution: total "dermis arthroplasty" of the knee joint. The early treatment of bone tumors combined with chemotherapy was another challenge on Ed's service at this time.

Ed usually talked fast during his presentations. My imitation of his presentation style did not work with my thick Hungarian accent. Again, Ed's advice proved to be invaluable to me: "Talk slowly and have lots of slides," he recommended. These tips were very helpful to me when I made combined orthopedic presentations in downtown Toronto in the presence of Drs. Dewar, Harris, Anderson, Salter, Pannel, and other leading orthopedic department chairmen.

Several times, Ed invited me to sail with him on his Nova Scotia schooner, which was moored at The Royal Canadian Yacht Club in Toronto. These outings would have been totally unattainable for me as a poor medical resident, and they exposed me to the entirely new, elite world of Torontonian society. As "Tom zee Bum," I also frequently was invited to be a dinner "guest" at Ed's house, where I got to know his lovely wife Joyce and their young toddler children. I will never forget, on several occasions in the Simmons's beautiful home, I met and socialized with Drs. Robert Mustard, Farmer, Lindsey, Salter, and others. What amazing experiences for a young intern and recent immigrant to Canada!

Ed also helped me to acquire the professional foundation that I needed to be accepted into the famous Gallie Course at the University of Toronto, and he provided me with the support that I needed to secure the opportunity to work as a research fellow in Dr. Bigelow's laboratory with Dr. Heimbecker at The Banting Institute in Toronto! This position was unforgettable and invaluable for me, since I had opportunities to meet the pioneers of heart surgery and other outstanding, internationally renowned surgeons: Drs. Henry Swan, Nauta, Dubost, Gerbode, Gordon

Murray, and others. Thanks to Ed!

After I began the Gallie Course at the University of Toronto, my professional life took another direction than Ed's, and I saw him less often. While I "struggled" through the rigorous surgical training program at the University of Toronto, the Gallie Course, Ed was developing new, pioneering, daring approaches to back surgery. He became internationally renowned, operating on patients coming from different continents and countries. Without a doubt his greatest pleasure was teaching, and he was selfless and tireless in his efforts to assist the trainees in orthopedic surgery. He helped them develop their specialty and careers. His teachings and interest in the postgraduate educations of orthopedic surgeons led to the development of the Simmons Orthopedic Society. The members of this Society later would become orthopedic chairpersons in various university training programs and leading surgeons in orthopedic surgery: Drs. Mike Simurda, Marv Tile, Joe Schatzker, and others.

Sailing with his family and sons—Ed Jr., Ian, and William—became Ed's personal outlet and serious hobby. He won numerous regatta trophies, while sailing on the Great Lakes under the ensigns of the Royal Canadian Yacht Club (R.C.Y.C.) of Toronto. During the 1970s, I often would run into Ed at the RCYC.

I have to digress at this point and eulogize Ed's lovely wife, Joyce. She was a steady supporter in all aspects of Ed's personal and professional lives. Until her early death, she reared his children and always stood behind him during the strenuous hours of his professional life.

During my hard times, when I was studying, doing clinical rotations, and performing research, the principles and guidance that Ed taught and gave me prevailed and worked. After I completed my training and moved to Buffalo, New York, to practice cardiothoracic surgery, Ed and I often met while we were sailing on Lake Ontario. For Ed, I always remained

"Tom zee Bum."

Ed's dynamic personality and professional accomplishments in orthopedic surgery during these years were without limits, and I suspect that he needed more "open space," growth outlets, and "better" working circumstances than those with which he was provided at Toronto East General Hospital.

One evening in the early 1980s, Ed telephoned me from Toronto to give me some interesting news. He stated that Dr. Eugene R. Mindell, the Chief of Orthopedic Surgery at the State University of New York at Buffalo, had contacted him looking for a promising candidate to fill the chief position in orthopedic surgery at the Buffalo General Hospital. Ed asked me about the hospital, the situation, and future possibilities there. At that time, our cardiac surgery practice in Buffalo was booming. We performed over 1,000 cases a year at the Buffalo General Hospital, and I thought that under the president of the hospital—Dr. Bill Kinard was the president—the future seemed very bright. I was delighted that in some ways, I could reciprocate at least a fraction of the favors and support with which Ed provided me during the early years of my training in Toronto. I enthusiastically campaigned for Ed to join the other surgeons and me operating at the Buffalo General Hospital and teaching medicine at the State University of New York at Buffalo.

Under Ed's guidance, the Orthopedic Department at Buffalo General Hospital started to flourish and became a truly international "institute" of back surgery. During these times at Buffalo General Hospital, Ed and I often mutually collaborated on presentations pertaining to spinal cord injuries, traumatic and vascular injuries of the spine, etc. Our respective departments became strong nuclei, increasing and spreading the scientific reputation of the Buffalo General Hospital. Ed and I also enjoyed skiing together during the yearly meeting of the Rocky Mountain Traumatological Society and sailing on Lake Ontario aboard his beautiful yacht, a Peterson 50. At our twenty-fifth anniversary cardiac surgery celebration in 1988, Ed served as the keynote speaker, describing the progressive scientific atmosphere of the Buffalo General Hospital as well as the attractions and qualities of life in Western New York.

Ed's scientific presentations always were perfect. He delivered them in impeccable English; they always were superbly organized, well-documented with slides and movies, and focused. In the 1990s, I traveled with Ed, Joyce, and Charlotte to Egypt, where Ed and I sailed Dragons in the Bay of Abukir (this was the area where Lord Nelson defeated the French fleet with Napoleon aboard in 1805). We also gave successful presentations at Cairo University, which, among other accomplishments, expanded the reputation of the Buffalo General Hospital.

On the Niagara River, where it empties into Lake Ontario, Youngstown, New York, became Ed's golden place of retirement. At his final home of pleasure there, he docked his yacht on the Niagara River. His wife Juanita provided him with loving care and affection.

It was one of the paradoxes of life—as they often happen—that Ed sustained a back fracture from falling downstairs in his home while trying to carry a huge Frederic Remington statue. The constant pain and neurological problems from the "Baker's" fracture he sustained shadowed the rest of his life and curtailed his sailing, traveling, and scientific involvements. Juanita's compassionate care and her constant attention helped to ease Ed's misery and sufferings.

The last time I talked to Juanita, when I was living in Greenwood, South Carolina early in 2009, I knew that the sunset of an outstanding surgeon, a great family patriarch, a true human being, and a great friend of five decades was sorrowfully and grievously approaching.

God Bless You, Ed!

APPENDIX 6
FESTSCHRIFT IN HONOR OF DR. WILFRED BIGELOW: HISTORICAL VIGNETTES INVOLVING "UNCLE BILL"

⁓

On the CTSNET.org, I read with great sadness that Dr. Wilfred Bigelow died on March 28, 2005, at the age of 91. After a half-century and many years away from Toronto, I still have extremely fond memories of working for Dr. Bigelow and for the great cardiac surgeons in Toronto.

I would like to send these remarks to you, being a disciple and colleague of Dr. Bigelow. You all still are in my fondest memories. During my one year at the Banting Institute under Dr. Ray Heimbecker and the half-year on the Cardiac Service at Toronto General Hospital in 1961, I got to know Dr. Bigelow and formed a close connection with him. The time I spent there has made a permanent imprint on me for the rest of my life.

Dr. Bigelow was a great surgeon, a great researcher, and the department chairman, who developed the cardiac service into an internationally renowned institution in Toronto. Last but not least, he was a true medical statesman.

I first met him at the Banting Institute in the research lab. At first sight of him, I was thoroughly overwhelmed and impressed by his personality.

Beyond research, at that time one of "my duties" was to go to the hospital's private patients' pavilion operating room and become familiar with the heart-lung machine. I was instructed to control the patient's temperature and adjust the temperature of the heat exchanger's hot and cold water in the pump circuit. The patient had to be cooled to twenty-eight centigrade and/or re-warmed to thirty-seven centigrade. I tried to do my duties with the utmost precision, just as well as any member of the team did. Small incidents colored those serious and somber days.

One day the pump technician got so involved with the perfusion of the patient that he fell asleep and fell to the floor; Dr. Bigelow looked back and remarked: "Denny, did you fall asleep?" I don't think there was any follow-up on this occurrence, but his voice was quite forbidding and scornful.

As a member of the heart team, one of my additional "duties" included driving up to Collingwood, Ontario with Ken, the head of the research lab, to collect stone-cold, frozen groundhogs from the groundhog farm and bring them back to the Banting Institute.

Dr. Bigelow supervised the lab and worked on his favorite research project: the hibernating hormone. He would look at me struggling to put dogs on the heart-lung machine, while I was trying to replace their tricuspid and mitral valves with fabricated aortic valve prostheses. He didn't say too much but always had a few good suggestions. At times, he escorted visitors from other pioneering centers through the lab, including Drs. Frank Gerbode, Henry Swan, and John Kirklin. I often thought that Dr. Bigelow appeared to be a humble escort, while the visitors like Dr. Swan and others looked and acted like the owners of the whole Banting Institute and the cardiac research lab.

I remember the day Dr. Bigelow showed his father, Dr. Bigelow Sr., from Brandon, Manitoba, Canada, around the laboratory. I realized instantly where Dr. Bigelow got the traits of "medical" blood and leadership.

The stream of international visitors from all over the world created a highly international and academic atmosphere and made the visits extremely colorful and memorable for all the residents. Some of the visitors included Dr. Niessen, from Switzerland; Drs. Boerema and Navratill, cardiac surgeons from Rotterdam; and Professor Charles

Dubost, from Paris. Lunches were provided for the "poor" residents like me. These visits were wonderful opportunities to spend time with outstanding, internationally renowned cardiac surgeons.

Dr. Bigelow's service was highly academic, but in a way, quite strict. Every time I had to do a presentation, I trembled and became somewhat incapacitated by my strong Hungarian accent.

Dr. Bigelow would repeatedly question: "What did you say?" Interestingly, Dr. Bigelow's attitude toward my accent was a permanent one, and after many, many years, whenever I met him, he always asked me: "What did you say?" In the spring of 2001, with my wife Charlotte, I attended a small gathering for Dr. Heimbecker, who at that time, had received and been honored with "The Order of Ontario" medal. When I introduced my wife to Dr. Bigelow—maybe because of my Hungarian origin—he asked my wife: "What did you say? Where are you from?"

Charlotte answered politely, "I am from Toronto, and my family has been Canadian for several generations."

In the early 1960s, I was a little bit reticent of Dr. Bigelow's policies. That was the time when three of the greatest North American heart surgeons—Drs. DeBakey, H. Swan, and W.G. Bigelow—were invited to Moscow by the Communist regime to advise "Dr. Petrowski," their host. Drs. DeBakey and Swan gave realistic reports about Russian cardiac surgery. Being a refugee from that same dictatorial system, I was disappointed to read Dr. Bigelow's evaluation of Russian cardiac surgery, including his political remarks.

Cardiac surgery carried a high risk of mortality. For both the patients and surgeons, it proved to be a very "stressful experience." The patient who underwent it had to make a huge decision about undergoing this type of surgery. When a patient died, it always caused an upset on the cardiac floor in the private patients' pavilion. One morning, Dr. Bigelow asked us whether we thought high-risk patients should be isolated prior to surgery, to avoid any disappointment when they did not return to the floor after surgery. The decision was unanimous: we said no. Patients had to realize the risks of cardiac surgery in the early 1960s.

The cardiac team was kept together by Dr. Bigelow's personality, charm, and graciousness. We first-year residents often were invited to cardiac parties. These events were the highlights of our training. As young residents, we could talk to these "divine individuals" on a one-to-one basis. Oftentimes there were some additional attractions at these parties: for example, one time Dr. Bigelow's gymnastically-inclined secretary performed acrobatics.

First call went to the junior resident during the day and/or night. One night, I received a call from the cardiac intensive care unit that a patient had developed fast atrial fibrillation. I digitalized the patient according to the protocol. The next morning, Dr. Bigelow took me aside and said it was beyond the range of my authority and ability to digitalize the patient without calling the appropriate cardiologist. I took this reprimand with humble acceptance. "Yes, sir." The next night when I was called again, as I had been instructed by Dr. Bigelow, I called the appropriate cardiologist, Dr. Herald Aldridge. His home telephone was busy at 2:00 a.m. and remained busy for at least twenty minutes. In a state of desperation, I called the police and asked them to go to Aldridge's home and awaken him. I apologized to him for this intrusion, and I received appropriate instructions from him to digitalize the patient, with a dosage very similar to what I had given the patient the day before. Aldridge still remembers the police incident, and we frequently chuckled about it when we met many decades after it occurred. He still remembers, since over the course of his career, he never again had been awakened by police to give an order at night to the cardiac unit.

Ever since, I am proud I strictly followed Dr. Bigelow's orders!

At times, I experienced hard times and had to "weather" the storms alone. One day, Dr. Bigelow summoned me to his office to ask me about a junior resident's performance; he solicited my recommendations regarding my colleague. Dr. Bigelow asked me if I would recommend him for the orthopedic training course. By that time, I had learned politics. I told Dr. Bigelow that I could not give a bad recommendation for my colleague and prevent him from further orthopedic training.

Shortly after this incident, Dr. Bigelow informed me that there was not an opening for me to be trained in cardiac surgery in Canada. This became the darkest day of my life.

In spite of this setback, I survived and maintained a cordial and friendly relationship with Dr. Bigelow, one of Canada's greatest surgeons. Thanks to one of the "Great Four," Dr. Heimbecker directed me to a position in St. Louis, Missouri, U.S.A., under Dr. Rollins C. Hanlon.

Dr. Bigelow never forgot me and mentioned me in his book titled *Cold Hearts*. He mentioned our mutual research with Dr. Heimbecker (1961) on "Ice Chip Cardioplegia." Later, he dedicated his other book on the *Mysterious Heparin* to me.

As years went by, each time I met him at different meetings, he eagerly asked me how things were going in Buffalo, New York, U.S.A., where I was practicing cardiac and thoracic surgery. I got the impression that even though I did not go through his cardiac post-graduate training, he still regarded me as one of his disciples. I appreciated and cherished my relationship with one of the great teachers and heart surgeons in Canada. We developed a common bond with unforgettable memories.

When I learned of Dr. Bigelow's death, I could not resist describing and sharing some of these historical vignettes in which I participated together with a great man, an outstanding surgeon, an inquisitive researcher, and a medical statesman.

Dr. Bigelow, I am sure God has blessed you. I will miss you.

Tom Lajos

BIBLIOGRAPHY

Applebaum, Anne. *The Iron Curtain: the Crushing of Eastern Europe, 1944-1956.* New York: Doubleday, Inc., 2012.

Gati, Charles. *Failed Illusions: Moscow, Washington, Budapest, and the 1956 Hungarian Revolt.* Stanford University Press, 2006.

Lajos, Ivan, Dr. *Germany's War Chances as Pictured in German Official Literature.* London: Victor Gollancz Ltd., 1939.

Lajos, Ivan, Dr. *Hungary's Responsibility in World War II.* Handwritten study. C.A. Macartney Collection. Bodleian Library, Oxford, UK. MSS Eng. c. C3291. Box 12, 183-232 portfolio, 1946.

Lajos, Ivan, Dr.. *Let Me Speak Up (Szotkerek): Evaluating the Gray Book ('Szurke Konyv.')* Budapest: Gergely R. Book Publisher, 1945.

Lajos, Ivan, Dr.. *(A Szurke Konyv) Németország háború̇s esélyei a német szakirodalom tükrében.* Budapest: Gergely R. Book Publisher, 1939.

Lajos, Thomas, Z. *Fallen to Tyranny: From Mauthausen to Gulag.* Bloomington, IN: AuthorHouse, 2012.

Muranyi, Gabor. *Egy epizodista foszerepe: Lajos Ivan tortenesz elete es halala.* Budapest: Noran Kiado KFT., 2006.

Parker, Robert. *Headquarters Budapest.* New York and Toronto: Farrar & Reinhart Inc., 1944.

Sebestyen, Victor. *Twelve Days: the Story of the 1956 Hungarian Revolution.* New York: Pantheon Books, 2006.

Tsetung, Mao. *Quotations from Chairman Mao Tsetung.* Peking: Foreign Languages Press, 1972.

NAME INDEX

Cooley, Denton, Chief Surgeon, Texas Heart Institute, Houston, TX, USA, 105, 164, 166, 206, 216

Cooper, Theodore, Assistant Secretary of Health, U.S. Department of Health, Education, and Welfare, 203

Creech, Arthur, Chief of Surgery, Tulane University, New Orleans, LA, USA, 207

Cross, Edward, medical doctor, Toronto East General Hospital, Ontario, Canada, 156

Csaky, Kalman, Count, Foreign Minister of Hungary, 27

Csanyi, Pal (Paul), husband of Ilus Lajos and brother-in-law of Ferenc Lajos, 17

Curteis, Ian Bayley, second husband of Lady Grantley (né Deirdre Listowel), 22

Daniel, Alexa, daughter of Erno and Katinka Daniel, 30, 31

Daniel, Erno, husband of Katinka Scipiades, pianist, conductor, Professor of Music, Santa Barbara, CA, USA, 30-31, 171

Daniel, Erno, Jr., cardiologist, son of Erno and Katinka Daniel, 30, 31

Daniel, Katinka (né Katinka Scipiades), see Scipiades, Katinka

DeBakey, Michael E., Chief of Surgery, Baylor and Methodist Hospitals, Houston, TX, USA, 179, 251

De Hevessy, George, scientist, Nobel Laureate, 57

Derose, Ms., operating room supervisor, Wellesley Hospital, Toronto, Ontario, Canada, 190

Dewar, Edward, Professor of Orthopedic Surgery, University of Toronto, Ontario, Canada, 158, 245

Doisy, Edward, Albert, Nobel Laureate, St. Louis University, St. Louis, MO, USA, 209

Donhoffer, Szilard, medical doctor, Professor of Patho-physiology, University of Pécs, Hungary, 88-89, 94, 96, 98-99, 101, 196

DuBost, Charles, Professor of Cardiac Surgery, Brusset, Paris, France, 163, 245, 251

Dulles, John Foster, U.S. Secretary of State, 114, 116, 235

Eber, Allan, Cistercian priest, teacher, 58

Eden, Sir Anthony, British Prime Minister, 114, 235

Egry, Jozsef, painter, 54-55

Eisenhower, Dwight, U.S. President, 114, 116, 126, 235

Eisert, Arpad, medical doctor, Professor, 100

Endredy, Vendel, Abbot of the Cistercian Order, Zirc, Hungary, 60

Ernst, Jeno, medical doctor, Professor, University of Pécs, Hungary, 83, 94, 95, 96

Farkas, Mihaly, communist accomplice, 240

Farmer, Chief of Surgery, The Hospital for Sick Children, Toronto, Ontario, Canada, 245

Farouk, Foud, Ismail, King of Egypt, 113

Felegyi, Roman, Cistercian priest, my principal, 59

Fermi, Enrico, Italian atomic scientist, 58

Festetics, George, Count, Keszthely, Hungary, 102

Forbath, Peter, cardiologist, St. Michael's Hospital, University of Toronto, Ontario, Canada, 105

Franz Ferdinand I, heir to the Austro-Hungarian monarchy, 79

Franz Joseph I, Kaiser of Austro-Hungarian monarchy, 40, 56, 79, 90, 111

Gaddafi, Muammar, dictator and ruler of Libya, 47, 116

Gamble, James, medical doctor, Professor, Harvard University, Boston, MA, USA, 96, 195

Gartha, medical doctor, 152

Gartha, Susanne, pediatrician, Toronto, Ontario, Canada, 152

Gati, Charles, Professor, Paul H. Nietze School of Advanced International Studies, The Johns Hopkins University, Washington, DC, USA, 232-238

Lajos, Laura, my daughter, 229

Lajos, Lenke (né Lenke Beke Bekehazy), wife of Ferenc Lajos, my paternal grandmother, 17,19,22,25,26,32,42,46,50,53,54,104,107,110,122,123,169

Lajos, Nagy, (The Great), Louis I, King of Hungary, 90, 91

Lajos, Paul, my son, 166, 170, 229

Lajos II, King of Hungary and King of Bohemia, 77

Lajos, Tamas, son of László Lajos and Agnes Lajos, my nephew, 129, 174, 175

Leger, Jacques, pathologist, friend, 154, 156-157

Lehotay, Judith, medical doctor, coroner, Erie County Medical Examiner, Buffalo, NY, U.S.A., 98

Lenin, Vladimir, Iljich, communist revolutionary, politician, and political theorist, 234

Lewis, John, Professor of Surgery, University of Chicago, IL, USA, 100, 161

Lewis, pediatric surgeon, St. Louis University, St. Louis, MO, USA, 206

Lincoln, Abraham, U. S. President, 208

Lindsey, W. R. N., plastic surgeon, Toronto East General Hospital, Ontario, Canada, 158, 245

Lissak, Kalman, medical doctor, Professor of Physiology, University of Pécs, Hungary, 96

Lister, Joseph, Sir., British surgeon and a pioneer of antiseptic surgery, London, UK, 143

Listowel, Deirdre, daughter of Lord and Lady Listowel, 3rd wife of Ian Bayley Curteis, 22

Listowel, Judith, Lady (né. Judith Márffy-Mantuano), daughter of Raoul Mantuano, married to William Hare, Fifth Earl of Listowel, 20, 21, 22

Listowel, William, Fifth Earl of, husband of Judith Márffy-Mantuano, 22

Littmann, Imre, cardiac surgeon, University of Budapest, Hungary,105, 140, 154, 164

Livingston, David, Scottish missionary and explorer, 22

Princip, Gavrilo, Serb Anarchist, assassin of Archduke Franz Ferdinand of Austria and Sophie, 79

Polanyi, Michael, scientist, Nobel Prize Winner, 57

Rajk, László, Hungarian Minister of Interior and Minister of Foreign Affairs, 63, 80

Rakosi, Mátyás, Deputy Prime Minister, Secretary of Hungarian Communist Party, 63, 80, 81, 83, 85, 121, 240

Rapp, surgeon, Toronto East General Hospital, Ontario, Canada, 152

Rauss, Károly, Professor of Microbiology, University of Pécs, Hungary, 96

Reagan, Ronald, U. S. President, 72, 234

Redward, Frank Gann, attache, British Legation, Budapest, Hungary, 54

Reh, Dezso, medical doctor, family friend, my guide to freedom, 123, 124, 125

Robertson, Charles, surgeon, Toronto East General Hospital, Ontario, Canada, 152, 187

Robicsek, Francis, Professor and Chief of Cardiac Surgery, Carolinas Heart Institute, Carolinas Medical Center, Charlotte, NC, USA, 105

Romhányi, Gyorgy, Professor of Pathology, University of Pécs, Hungary, 94, 98

Roosevelt, Franklin Delano, U.S. President, 13, 66, 114

Ross, Donald, Sir, Chief of Cardiac Surgery, London, England, UK, 207

Rozsnyai, Zoltan, conductor, 38

Salter, Robert, Chief of Orthopedics, The Hospital for Sick Children, Toronto, Ontario, Canada, 158, 245

Sandiford, medical doctor, Secretary of the British Medical Association, London, UK, 140

Sanford, Denny, pump technician, 165, 250

Santha, Oliver, Reverend, 60

Saperstein, Wolf, cardiac surgeon, 178

Sass-Kortsak, Andrew, medical doctor, The Hospital for Sick Children, Toronto, Ontario, Canada, 97, 194-195

Savoy, Eugene, Prince of, Commander of the European Army against the Turks, 77

Sawyer, Department of Medicine, St. Michael's Hospital, Toronto, Ontario, Canada, 155, 159

Scala, Sam, medical doctor, 157

Schatzker, Joseph, Chief of Orthopedic Surgery, Wellesley Hospital, Toronto, Ontario, Canada, 246

Schmidt, Lajos, Professor of Surgery, University of Pécs Medical School, Pécs, Hungary, 96

Schumacher, Harry, Chief of Surgery, Indiana University, IN, USA, 203

Schuschnigg, Kurt, President of Austria, before the Anschluss, 209

Schweiss, John, Chief of Anesthesia, St. Louis University, St. Louis, MO, USA, 206

Scipiades, Elemer, Jr., son of Professor Elemer Scipiades, medical doctor, 30

Scipiades, Elemer, Professor of Obstetrics and Gynecology, University of Pécs, Hungary, 23, 29-30, 37, 44

Scipiades, Katinka (married name Mrs. Katinka Daniel), daughter of Professor Elemer Scipiades, 30-31, 171

Scipiades, Nora, daughter of Professor Elemer Scipiades, 30

Scott, Catherine, sister of Charlotte Lajos, 170, 198

Semmelweiss, Ignaz, Professor of Obstetrics and Gynecology, discoverer of Puerperal Sepsis, Budapest, Hungary, 143

Shiptar, Endre, teacher, 59

Shumway, Norman, Professor of Cardiac Surgery, Stanford University, Palo Alto, CA, USA, 203

Siegel, John, Chief of Surgery, Buffalo General Hospital, Buffalo, NY, USA, 98

Sigray, Antal, Count, representative of Karoly IV, 43

Simmons, Edward H., friend, mentor, Chief, Orthopedic Surgery, Buffalo General Hospital, Buffalo, NY, USA, 153, 155, 157-158, 160, 212, 244-248

Simurda, Michael, Chief of Orthopedic Surgery, Queen's University, Kingston, Ontario, Canada, 246

Sirak, Howard, cardiac surgeon, Ohio State University Hospitals, Columbus, OH, USA, 214-215, 216

Sissi (Elisabeth), Kaiserin, Empress of Austria and Queen of Hungary, wife of Emperor Franz Joseph I, 90

Sones, Mason, F., Head of Catheter Laboratory, Cleveland Clinic Foundation, Cleveland, OH, USA, 182

Sophie Ferdinand, wife of Franz Ferdinand I, 79

Soutar, H., medical doctor, 218

Spivak, Manny, Chief Resident of Obstetrics and Gynecology, Toronto General Hospital, Ontario, Canada, 187

Stalin, (Djugasvili) Joseph, leader of the USSR, 12, 13, 26, 47, 65, 66, 67, 68, 73, 75, 76, 78, 81, 83, 85, 107, 108, 114, 121, 240, 242

Starr, Albert, cardiac surgeon, inventor of Starr-Edwards heart valve, University of Oregon, OR, USA, 167

Steel, John, Professor, Editor, Annals of Thoracic Surgery, 218

Sterns, Ernie, surgeon, Queens University, Kingston, Ontario, Canada, 185, 186, 191, 225

Stevens, John, Christopher, U.S. Ambassador to Libya, 116

Suleiman the Great, Turkish Sheikh, Sultan of the Ottoman Empire, 1520-1566, 77

Suslov, Michael, Soviet Deputy, communist party ideologist, 112, 113, 234, 235

Todd, Ian, Chief Resident, Urology, Sunnybrook Health Sciences Centre, Toronto, Ontario, Canada, 187

Togut, Allen, resident in Thoracic Surgery, Ohio State University Hospital Columbus, OH, USA, 213-214

Tovie, Bruce, Division Head, General Surgery, Toronto General Hospital, Ontario, Canada, 186, 191

Trimble, A., Chief Resident, Cardiac Surgery, Toronto General Hospital, Ontario, Canada, 162, 163

Tzagournis, M., Dean, Ohio State University, Columbus, OH, USA, 217

Tsetung, Mao, Chairman, China, 76, 77, 236

Voroshilov, Kliment Yefremovich, Soviet Marshal, 80

Vozoris, James, Chief Resident, General Surgery, Toronto East General Hospital, Ontario, Canada, 152

Walker, anesthesiologist, Whipps Cross Hospital, London E. 11, England, UK, 143

Wallenberg, Raoul, Swedish diplomat, 27-28, 85

Waters, Neal, Chief of Surgery, Wellesley Hospital, Toronto, Ontario, Canada, 190, 191, 192

Wende, Janos, medical doctor, 79

Wigner, Eugene, atomic scientist, Nobel Prize winner, 57

Williams, Bud, Chief Resident, General Surgery, Toronto East General Hospital, Ontario, Canada, 152

Willman, Vallee, Chief of Surgery, St. Louis University, St. Louis, MO, USA, 202, 204, 211, 212

Wilson, Woodrow, U.S. President, 66